ness for Life

Fitness for Life
Exercises for People Over 50

THEODORE BERLAND

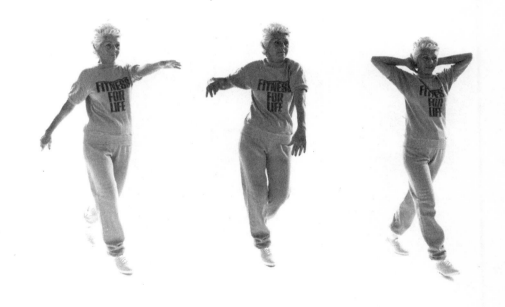

An AARP Book
published by
American Association of Retired Persons, Washington, D.C.
Scott, Foresman and Company, Lifelong Learning Division,
Glenview, Illinois

The following organizations kindly provided models to illustrate many of the exercises in this book:

> The Multiplex Fitness Club for Men and Women, Deerfield, Illinois
> Casa Central, Chicago, Illinois
> The White Crane Tai Chi Club and White Crane Senior Health Center at Illinois Masonic Hospital, Chicago, Illinois

Library of Congress Cataloging in Publication Data

Berland, Theodore, 1929–
    Fitness for life.

    Bibliography: p.
    Includes index.
    1. Exercise for the aged.   2. Physical fitness
for the aged.   I. Title.
RA781.B434   1986   613.7'1'0240565   85-18267
ISBN 0-673-24812-7

AARP Books is an educational and public service project of the American Association of Retired Persons, which, with a membership of 20 million, is the largest association of persons fifty and over in the world today. Founded in 1958, AARP provides older Americans with a wide range of membership programs and services, including legislative representation at both federal and state levels. For further information about additional association activities, write to AARP, 1909 K Street, N.W., Washington, DC 20049.

Books by Theodore Berland

The Scientific Life
Your Children's Teeth
The Fight for Quiet
The Fitness Fact Book
Rating the Diets
The Acupuncture Diet
After the Diet . . . Then What?
The Doctor's Calories-Plus Diet
The Dieter's Almanac
Living With Your Ulcer
Living With Your Bad Back
Living With Your Bronchitis and Emphysema
Living With Your Eye Operation
Living With Your Colitis, Hemorrhoids, and Related Disorders
Living With Your Allergies and Asthma

For Carol

Contents

Foreword

There have been significant changes in the American lifestyle in the past fifty years. Automobiles, elevators, and a vast array of laborsaving devices have significantly reduced the physical exertion required in the workplace. Television viewing has replaced less-sedentary leisure activities. Obesity has replaced malnutrition as a dietary concern. Recently, however, many Americans have become conscious of the vital role played by exercise and proper nutrition in their physical and mental well-being. *Fitness for Life* will have the most casual reader joining this group. The elements of a successful exercise program are explained, and the building blocks to tailor an individualized program are provided. Relaxation and diet, as important complements to exercise, are addressed. The book is focused for people over fifty, but it is a clarion call to readers of all ages to make a personal commitment to physical fitness—for life.

GEORGE ALLEN
Chairman
President's Council on Physical
Fitness and Sports

Preface

This book is designed to meet the need of the swelling ranks of citizens who are fifty years of age and older, who have been sedentary for most of their lives, and who have a new feeling that the quality of their lives may depend on the measure of their fitness.

In order to provide a full perspective of the role of exercise in functional fitness, the author sought information from a wide range of authoritative sources.

Among the institutions that provided important information were the President's Council on Physical Fitness and Sports and the National Association for Human Development.

Published works such as textbooks on the physiology of exercise and guides to exercise were also used as sources. A bibliography at the end of the book indicates the major published sources used as references, should you wish, or should your doctor wish, in-depth information.

In addition, much of the information and advice presented here comes from the writings and conversations of fourteen experts and represents a consensus of their findings and judgment, rather than that of any individual. The author wishes to acknowledge with thanks their time, talent, advice, and permission to be quoted. The author also wishes to emphasize that this book is solely his responsibility so that any errors of fact or judgment are his and are in no way the responsibility of any expert he spoke with or quoted.

The experts:

Kenneth H. Cooper, M.D., M.P.H. Director of the Aerobic Center, Dallas. Formerly with the U.S.A.F. Medical Corps. Founder of the aerobics system that is the official fitness program of the U.S.A.F., U.S. Navy, and the Royal Canadian Air Force. Author of *Aerobics* and four other books.

Charles B. Corbin, Ph.D. Professor of physical education, Arizona State University. Author of *Concepts in Physical Education* and *A Textbook of Motor Development*.

David E. Corbin, Ph.D. Assistant professor in the School of Health, Physical Education and Recreation, University of Nebraska at Omaha. Coauthor of *Reach for It!*

Josie Metal-Corbin, M.Ed. Assistant professor in the School of Health, Physical Education and Recreation at the University of Nebraska at Omaha. Coauthor of *Reach for It!*

Herbert A. deVries, Ph.D. Director of the Physiology of Exercise Laboratory at the Andrus Gerontology Center at the University of Southern California. Author of *Fitness After 50* and four textbooks on health and exercise.

Lilias Folan, Cincinnati. Author of *Yoga and Your Life* and perhaps the best-known yoga teacher in the United States, having appeared regularly on her own television program syndicated to 200 public television stations.

Saul S. Haskell, M.D. Attending physician, Department of Orthopedic Surgery, and director of the Sports Medicine Program, Michael Reese Hospital and Medical Center, Chicago.

David K. Leslie, Ph.D. Professor of physical education, University of Iowa. Coauthor of *Exercises for the Elderly*.

Henry S. Miller, M.D. Medical director, Cardiac Rehabilitation Program, Wake Forest University; Professor of Medicine, Bowman Gray School of Medicine.

Gabe Mirkin, M.D. Assistant professor of sports medicine, University of Maryland. Author of *The Sportsmedicine Book* and *Getting Thin*. Columnist, *New York Times;* commentator, CBS Radio.

Gail Schreiber, R.N. Stanford University Arthritis Program.

Robert R. Spackman, Jr., M.S., R.P.T. Associate professor, Physical Education, Southern Illinois University, Carbondale. Author of *Conditioning for Senior Citizens*.

Karl Stoedefalke, Ph.D. Professor of Health, Physical Education and Recreation, The Pennsylvania State University.

Wilma York, R.N., M.S. Consultant to Marin Senior Coordinating Council, San Rafael, California. Former professor at Mankato State University and the University of Nevada.

Introduction

Previously published books on exercises for middle-aged and older persons have addressed the reader as aged and infirm and have often assumed that there was little physical improvement possible. In these last years of the twentieth century, this approach has been proven misguided and erroneous.

While physical fitness is affected by a physical aging component, it is relatively minor. The major components of physical fitness at any age are the amounts and kinds of exercise that are undertaken and maintained on a regular basis.

This book is dedicated to getting persons who have been inactive into the kind of physical condition that will enable them to undertake the kinds of activities they wish. For persons who have been active for many years, this book can provide a guide for lifting themselves to even higher plateaus of physical fitness so that they can—should they choose—compete in active sports such as swimming and running.

The chapters that follow contain details of specific components of the values of exercise: cardiovascular fitness, flexibility, muscle strength and endurance, and leanness. Also there are details, with photographs, of exercises at four levels of intensity, as well as information and advice to help you assess your own fitness level and plan your individual exercise program. There is also advice on sports so you can see whether any are for you, and, if so, which are best. Another chapter details techniques of relaxation and explains that rest and relaxation are essential to a Fitness for Life program. Later in the book there is advice on choosing exercise equipment and on the pros and cons of joining a health club. Special techniques for preventing pain, sports injuries, and illnesses associated with exercise are offered also, as well as advice on first-aid treatment for pain, injuries, and illnesses that were not prevented.

The heart of the book is its four-part program of exercises and activities, each leading to a higher level of fitness. What level of fitness you should seek to attain is up to you. Your decision should hinge on how you want to live your life and what you want to do.

Fitness here means the ability to move and function within your physical limitations. You can reach one level of fitness and stay there. Or, you can start at the lowest level of exercises, master it, and move up to the next level, and, perhaps to the highest, and thus achieve a level of maximum fitness. You can climb as many levels as you like and physically can.

The point is this: You can do it—no matter your age. This book is dedicated to that proposition.

1 Fitness for Function

When you were very young, exercise was nice to do, and fitness was admirable to achieve.

Now, exercise must be regular, and fitness must be continuous.

The truth is that while fitness is optional in childhood, it is important for good health in adulthood.

A disposable part of your lifestyle when you were younger, exercise must be an integral part of your lifestyle now that you are mature.

Ideally, you should have been exercising continually from youth. And that is a good message for younger persons. But you are what you are now. According to surveys, most persons fifty and older do not exercise regularly. But research indicates that they can still benefit if they start an exercise program and stick to it.

However, before you consider an exercise program, you should consult with your physician so that your physical limitations can be accurately assessed. Then you will know which kinds of activities, and at what intensity level, you can safely perform.

Your physician will consider your past history of health and disease as well as your current condition and any infirmity you may have and will take into account the effects of any medications you may be taking. The doctor may want to take some tests, such as a stress test and lung function tests, in order to more precisely evaluate your exercise limitations.

The examination should be as thorough as necessary to enable your doctor to discover any and all hidden defects in your heart, blood circulation, and respiratory system and any degree of arthritis that limits motions of your joints. The stress test is usually no more than an electrocardiogram (ECG) taken during some measured exercise, most often on a treadmill or stationary cycle. Often, exhaled breath is simultaneously analyzed for carbon dioxide content as a measure of your metabolism and respiration. The stress test is called that because it is

Too many believe that one should exercise until one is 20 to 25 years and then they have enough fitness built in to last the next 50 years. Physical fitness lasts about three weeks. Exercise isn't for kids as most people believe. Exercise is for everyone over 21 years, the more over 21, the more exercise one needs.
—"Doc" Spackman, Trainer

3

designed to stress the body to a safe but crucial level so as to reveal irregularities that would not be likely to show up in tests taken when you are at rest.

Once your physician has determined your degree of fitness and your limitations, he or she can consult with you on the details of your planned exercise program; then you can get started.

If you have not kept in shape over the years, you have a lot of catching up to do.

But don't feel guilty or alone. Many people are in the same situation. It is easy to see how it happened. Most likely, the reduction in your physical activity followed two attitudes that developed imperceptibly over the years.

First of all, there was your acceptance of mechanization. You grew up during those years when laborsaving devices became wonderfully ubiquitous in home and workplace. During your lifetime, society used less and less muscle power as it went, for example, from hand-operated eggbeaters to electric mixers in the kitchen, from hand mowers to power mowers on the lawn, and from hand-operated to pneumatic-powered wrenches in the shop. In a century, our society converted from muscle power to machine power, and the main source of energy changed from food for muscles to coal, oil, gas, electricity, and atomic energy for machines. The result is that you were seduced by the ease of pushing a button. You sat back and let the mechanisms and the electronics do all the work for you.

This attitude spared you sweating and doing chores, but it also significantly reduced the level of your physical activity well below any limitations of health.

The other attitude that hindered your physical activities was the expectation that physical decline was inevitable, and that it accelerated with age. You believed the predominant image of the "middle-aged" and "old" displayed in novels, movies, and other popular communication media as that of decrepit, dried-out men and women who spend their days and nights in rocking chairs.

How wrong those attitudes are! The reality of middle-aged and older persons is quite different from the popular attitudes and images. Even advanced age, by itself, is no longer a barrier to an active life.

The variety of individual capacities and capabilities among human beings is incredibly wide. We are supposed to be politically equal, but we are physiologically unique, each with his or her own distinct strengths and weaknesses. Also, each person (again, at any age) has certain constitutional limitations. Still, within your limitations you can rely more on your strengths than on your weaknesses. Physical impairments and chronic disease (at any age) merely limit the *range* of a person's activity, not the person's ability to be active.

You can be more physically active than you are now, perhaps even more active than you dared hope. In fact, you *must be* more active for your own good.

You can fulfill your potential for functioning better, for being able to do more, by exercising. That's what fitness for function means—being fit enough to do what you want to do.

Exercising regularly doesn't mean you have to try to become a "jock" and train like an athlete. This does not mean that you have to tax your heart, lungs, and joints. Also, you do not have to take any risks, and you do not have to experience pain as you exercise.

It does mean that you can follow a program of exercise that respects your limitations and weaknesses as it expands your ability to function by amplifying your strengths and endurance.

Exercise can help you live your life to its fullest. This is true no matter your age, condition, and present lifestyle. Exercise can help the active as well as the sedentary, the very healthy as well as the not so healthy. It can help those who have been lucky enough to come through life unscathed thus far by major illness or trauma. It also can help those with chronic diseases: the arthritic, the diabetic, the heart patient, the stroke victim, and the cancer patient.

Exercise can help you—no matter your condition or disease—by allowing you to do more and to get more out of life. Then you will learn that aging is not so much a function of years as it is a function of fitness—or lack of it. The better your functional fitness, the younger you will be, the younger you will act, and the younger you will appear.

Exercise offers these twenty-two benefits.

- improved cardiovascular fitness
- improved lung capacity
- improved capacity for work
- improved fatigue level
- improved endurance
- improved vigor
- improved resistance against diseases
- improved metabolism
- improved digestion
- improved bowel function
- improved bone mass and strength
- improved joint flexibility
- improved neuromuscular coordination and skills
- improved relaxation

- improved sleep
- improved sexual function
- improved figure
- improved general appearance
- improved feeling of well-being
- improved attitude
- improved ability to cope with stress
- improved mood

Even if you have never exercised before, starting now will do much to slow the processes of physical deterioration. Fitness that comes with exercising can even reverse some of the deterioration that is due not to aging but to disuse.

For instance, it used to be assumed that aging alone slowed reflexes and interfered with coordination. This was exemplified by the older person's slow, bent walk and poor balance.

Actually, these are mainly the effects of lack of use of muscles and the nerves that control them and of a loss of the simple pleasure of being able to move. Some of this effect is due to a psychological distortion of body image, which sets up a vicious cycle. You see yourself as slow and bent, and soon you behave that way. Then your body accustoms itself to the inactivity. Finally, you are as you envisioned yourself. The expectation is fulfilled.

With disuse, muscles shrink, shorten, and weaken. With no demands placed upon them, blood vessels lose their elasticity as their inner surfaces narrow, thus restricting blood flow. The heart responds similarly.

The body and its components respond to stimulation. They are there to serve, to be used. Even persons who have suffered severe trauma or stroke know that effort and use can work wonders to bring back function of both limbs and intellect. Study after study has shown that exercise—even mild exercise—can restore much of the strength of muscles and improve the functioning of the nervous system, the respiratory system, and the cardiovascular system.

In short, physical activity can reverse much of that deterioration of the body that cavalierly used to be ascribed to old age, and it can delay aging changes. While exercise alone cannot instantly restore all the ravages of trauma and disease, a well-planned program of exercise can go a long way toward helping bring back function. At the same time, it can vastly improve disease-free and trauma-free parts of the body.

Every single improvement in your physical condition will come only with effort. And it will not come suddenly. It will come only after you have been exercising for a while. You will gradually feel better, but do not expect to feel wonderful right away. In fact, you may experience some muscle soreness for the first few weeks, even though you are in good health and have been doing the exercises properly and regularly. This soreness is good. It is an indication that your muscles are responding and that they will soon be a bit stronger and will have an increment more endurance than before you started the exercises. So you are going to have to be patient of your progress and tolerant of your body's sometimes slow but positive responsiveness to the challenge of exercise.

As you cannot expect to have immediate results, so you cannot expect to plunge into exercise with full intensity. Perhaps young people can do that and not suffer harm to their bodies. However, older persons must approach exercise more cautiously and systematically. As you'll see in the chapters that follow, you will have to start slowly—first with motions for limbering up muscles and joints (which are barely exercises), then mild stretches, then mild exercises.

If you have never exercised, or have not exercised in a long time, you may be apprehensive about starting now, at this stage of life. Such apprehension, and even fear, are to be expected. You don't want to suffer pain, and you certainly don't want to do anything that will injure yourself. That's why the exercises offered here are presented in a stepped fashion—starting with the very mild and allowing you to work up in intensity, if you wish and if your doctor agrees that you should do so. Also, the exercises presented here remain at the level of motion and intensity that best suits you and your condition.

Whatever your individual exercise program, you should experience an improvement in your fitness that will enable you to do more than you were able to do before.

The only way to be more active than you are now is to become more active—to do more. If you can jog, fine. If you can walk, fine. If you can swim, fine. Every bit of additional activity will beget yet more activity. Move a little more now and in a little while you will be able to function even better.

The concept is that simple. But there are two hitches:

1. You are the one who has to exercise; no one can do it for you.

2. You have to exercise regularly, faithfully, and as long as you live (of course, exercising regularly may help you live longer).

Finally, you have to be realistic about exercise. While most of this book emphasizes what exercise can do for you positively, you should be aware that exercise can do things to you negatively. You should not be exercising because it is the thing to do these days. Rather, exercise should serve a purpose—to help you do the things you want to do, or do better, in your daily life. That means that some exercises are appropriate, and some are not.

Exercise *can* harm you when you are not properly prepared, when you have physical ailments, and when you do too much too fast.

Any harm happens more readily to bodies that are out of shape. If yours is one of them, no matter your age, it is crucial that you see your physician, do the Functional Fitness Self-Assessment to learn about your fitness level, and undertake only those exercises that will help you—and only at the level at which you should be entering an exercise program.

2 Fitness and Health

No respectable doctor will guarantee that you will live *longer* if you are fit. But just about every doctor will tell you that you will live *better* if you are fit. "Better" means not only being able to function as you wish, and do what you want to do, but also being able to function for many more days a year than the unfit, simply because you will be healthier.

Whether or not exercise can hold off death, it most certainly can hold off the normal effects of aging. Many of these effects are the result of losing the war with gravity. You know you are losing that war when your abdomen protrudes, your flesh sags, your shoulders droop, your joints stiffen, and your posture is bent.

There is, in other words, a direct relationship between fitness and health. You might regard it as a ratio: the better your fitness, the better your health. And the better your health, the better you feel, the better you look, and the more you can do.

Every new level of fitness that you achieve will help your health. Properly done and consistently done, exercises need not be strenuous or painful. Yet they will help you achieve and maintain the level of fitness that can best help you function in your style of life. The bodily benefits of fitness are many and include a better figure, an improved general look, and a more favorable disposition. If you are still working, you will notice improved performance and productivity.

Because it is such a big benefit of exercise, cardiovascular fitness is discussed in detail in another chapter. This chapter will detail all health benefits, as well as some of the health cautions that some conditions and diseases dictate you observe.

AMA's Health Benefits

The Council on Scientific Affairs of the American Medical Association (AMA) in the summer of 1984 issued a report, endorsed by the

Much of the physical frailty attributed to aging is actually the result of muscular disuse and poor diet. And, many such problems can be halted, or even reversed, through proper eating habits and a regular exercise program to improve cardiovascular endurance, muscle strength, and flexibility.
—Pep Up Your Life: A Fitness Book for Seniors

9

AMA House of Delegates, which noted that "many of the changes in body structure and function commonly attributed to aging can be retarded by an active exercise program." The so-called effects of aging are actually biological alterations that come with inactivity and disuse. Furthermore, it was stated that "physical activity will also improve the older person's psychological image and contribute to improved mental health."

The report noted the following physiological and emotional benefits of exercise.

- improved cardiorespiratory conditioning
- improved metabolic and endocrine functions, with an increased ability to handle stress
- increased aerobic capacity, with an increase in the ability of the blood to absorb and transport oxygen to the tissues, which have an increased ability to absorb oxygen
- increased capacity to do physical work
- prevention of bone loss (osteoporosis) and an increase in bone mass
- lower percentage of body fat and an increase in lean body mass
- overall better general health rating
- better capacity to cope with daily environmental hazards that come with such life activities as walking and driving an automobile
- faster reaction times and movements
- improved unity of mind and body, which comes with an improved self-image and a more positive approach toward life

Physicians should "encourage all their patients to establish an exercise program as a lifetime commitment in preparation for their later years," said the AMA council report. "Advancing age should not preclude regular exercise. Indeed, it is at least as important for the older person to engage in a suitable exercise program under medical supervision as it is for the younger, more vigorous individual."

Additional Health Benefits

Other reports have listed additional health benefits of exercise. Among them are these:

- reduction of triglycerides and cholesterol in the blood
- increased peripheral circulation

- lowered resting heart rate
- increased heart efficiency
- lowered blood pressure
- increased lung capacity
- improved physical coordination
- enhancement of relaxation
- reduction of anxiety and tension conditions such as headache, backache, and insomnia

Benefits of exercise in two specific conditions, diabetes and arthritis, are detailed below.

Diabetes

Exercise lowers blood sugar by improving insulin sensitivity. If you are a diabetic, this means that on days you exercise, you probably can eat more food on less insulin than on days you don't exercise.

Exercise also lowers LDL (low-density lipoprotein) cholesterol, the substance in blood that clogs arteries and so causes heart attack and stroke. Insulin-dependent diabetics suffer a higher than normal incidence of these cardiovascular diseases. In large part this is because they have abnormally high LDL cholesterol levels in their blood. So, by lowering LDL cholesterol levels, exercise helps protect diabetics against such diseases.

The exercise effect applies not only to Type I, or *insulin-dependent,* diabetes but also to Type II, which is controlled solely by diet or by a program of diet and oral medication.

However, if you have diabetes, do *not* change your diet or your medication dosage when you start exercising until you check with your doctor. Exercise or no, you still have to keep your food intake and medication in balance to maintain good health.

Arthritis

Exercise can help break the vicious cycle in which the pain and swelling of arthritis discourages movement of your joints. The continued disuse, in turn, leads to shrinking and weakening of muscles around the joints, which further limits joint motion and causes more muscle atrophy, and so on.

Often you can regain a significant portion of a joint's motion by exercising, especially stretching and strengthening. In such instances, there may be a bit of pain at first, but the more consistent you are in exercising the afflicted joint, the easier it will be to move the joint the next time. Also, the surrounding muscles will stay stronger and thus help decrease the likelihood of joint contraction, disability, and deformity.

Note these cautions.

- Exercise each involved joint every day.
- Move slowly and gently.
- Don't exercise the first thing in the morning, when you are likely to be stiff.
- Don't exercise beyond the point of pain.

Another important caution: If the joint is hot and inflamed, do not exercise it. In this condition, the joint can be hurt rather than helped, or, in medical terms, the acute arthritis can be exacerbated.

Time Is of the Essence

As you can see, the health benefits of exercise are many—and important. But the benefits are as fleeting or as permanent as is your commitment to exercise and fitness. That is because there are two time factors in fitness:

1. It is true that the earlier in life you achieve maximum fitness, the more likely it is that you will be healthy in youth and after, into the middle and older years. However, you should not be discouraged if you are just now getting around to putting yourself in shape. The adage, Better late than never, applies. If you start your program now, you can at least hang on to what you have; more likely, you will improve your fitness and health. If you do nothing, your fitness level and your health may deteriorate—and more quickly than you imagine.

2. Fitness is temporary, and its health benefits are temporary. That is, if you reach a high plateau of fitness and health, you will stay at that height only as long as you exercise. Both your fitness and your health will slip down the mesa like rainwater once you discontinue your exercise program.

The message is clear: exercise to get in shape and stay in shape. Thus can you improve your health and maintain it. Thus can you enjoy life and keep living a fuller one.

3 Assessing Your Fitness

Your fitness program is designed to close the gap between what you are and what you want to be, no matter the present circumstances of your life. But even before you start thinking about putting together a personal program of Fitness for Life, you have to know what base you are operating from. In designing a fitness program for yourself, you must first know your present level of fitness and then decide what level of fitness you want to work toward.

Thus, assessing your fitness is the first order of business. This chapter offers the Functional Fitness Self-Assessment, which enables you to score yourself on several tests in order to help you find your fitness level. You can build your fitness program upon this base to achieve the level of functional fitness you desire.

A note of caution: Do only what you can do easily on the physical parts of the assessment. Don't strain yourself or otherwise tax your body to show how fit you are. If you do, you may pay for it later.

Please bear in mind that this quick assessment is essentially for persons who are healthy or have but minor physical impairments. The assessment is in no way a substitute for a complete physical examination by your doctor. That is a must.

Again, be cautious as you go through this self-assessment. The best way to complete it is to have a friend help and score you. If that person is a "fitness buddy" who is also working on a personal fitness program, all the better!

Assessing Your Body

The Functional Fitness Self-Assessment essentially evaluates four areas of fitness: flexibility, muscle strength, endurance, and body fat. You'll score yourself at the conclusion of your assessment of each of these four major areas and then compute a total that will give you an overall Functional Fitness Self-Assessment score.

In a technical sense, physical fitness can be viewed as a measure of the body's strength, stamina, and flexibility. In more meaningful personal terms, it is a reflection of your ability to work with vigor and pleasure, without undue fatigue, with energy left for enjoying hobbies and recreational activities, and for meeting unforeseen emergencies. It relates to how you look and feel—and, because the body is not a compartment separate from the mind, it relates to how you feel mentally as well as physically.
—President's Council on Physical Fitness and Sports

13

Before you attempt any of the exercises on the assessment, warm up by walking around for five minutes, then slowly bending your trunk sideways and forward and back. As you take each test, do your best, but don't overdo.

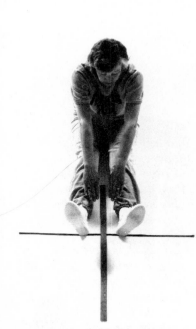

1. Trunk Stretch. Sit on the floor or a mat or bed so that your legs are extended straight before you, with heels about five inches apart. Mark with tape (or some other way) a line from heel to heel. Take a yardstick and line it up between your legs so that the fifteen-inch mark is at the line and the 0-inch end is closest to your crotch. The test is performed by slowly reaching your hands forward as far as you can. Be sure you do not jerk. Just stretch forward and place your fingertips on the yardstick and measure. Do this three times and record the best (farthest) stretch. If you are a male-female fitness buddy team, you may notice that the woman is more flexible than the man. That's normal; females generally are more supple than males at every stage of life. Here's how to score your performance.

Above 17 inches	5 points
15 to 17 inches	4 points
12 to 14 inches	3 points
9 to 11 inches	2 points
Below 9 inches	1 point

2. Hip Bend. Keep the yardstick from the previous test. Stand straight; then bend forward at the hips. Try to position your back parallel to the floor. Slowly straighten up. Take the yardstick. Extend your arms in front of you so that the yardstick, in both hands, is parallel to the floor. Now bend forward again, this time keeping your extended arms in front of you. With your back bent forward as parallel to the

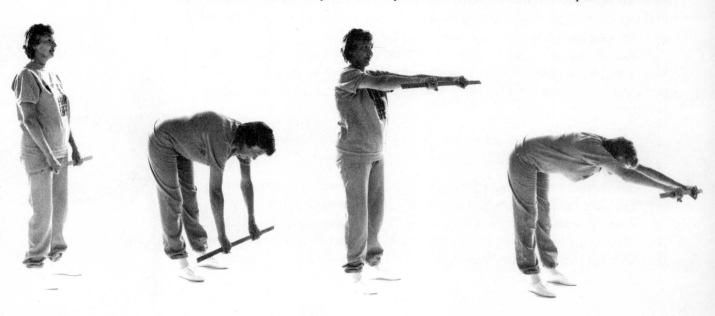

floor as it can be, see how high you can raise the yardstick. Then score yourself as follows:

Yardstick above eye level	5 points
Yardstick at eye level	4 points
Yardstick just below eye level	3 points
Yardstick well below eye level	2 points
Yardstick closer to knees than eyes	1 point

3. Toe Touch.   From a standing position, bend at the hips and reach for your toes. This will produce stretching, so stop and lift up a bit if you feel any pain. Move smoothly, not in jerky motions. Here's how to score yourself.

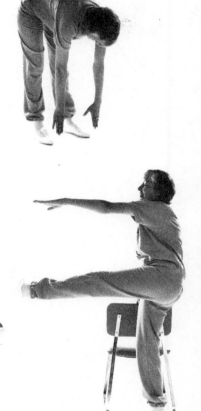

Fingertips on toes	5 points
Fingertips on ankles	4 points
Fingertips on lower shins	3 points
Fingertips on upper shins	2 points
Fingertips on knees	1 point

4. Leg Kick.   With one hand holding a chair or pressing against a wall, lift your straightened left leg in front of you, as parallel to the floor as you can get it. Extend your free arm above your leg, and try to touch your fingertips with your toes. Do the left leg three times and then the right leg three times, and score yourself with the best of the six attempts, as follows:

Toes touching fingertips	5 points
Toes 6 inches below fingertips	4 points
Toes 12 inches below fingertips	3 points
Toes 18 inches below fingertips	2 points
Toes 24 inches below fingertips	1 point

5. Side Kick.   This is similar to the leg kick, except that you do this to the side, lifting as high as you can, first the left leg, then the right, three times each. Take the best of the six kicks to score yourself.

Toes touching fingertips	5 points
Toes 6 inches below fingertips	4 points
Toes 12 inches below fingertips	3 points
Toes 18 inches below fingertips	2 points
Toes 24 inches below fingertips	1 point

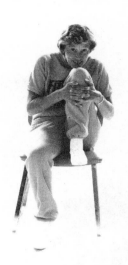

6. Knee Squeeze.   Sitting in a chair, raise one leg as high as you can, keeping the knee bent without causing any pain. The idea is to pull the bent leg as close to your chest as it will go. It's all right to use your arms and hands (smoothly, not with any jerky motion) to pull the leg up. Score yourself.

Knee touching chin	5 points
Knee 3 inches from chin	4 points
Knee 6 inches from chin	3 points
Knee 9 inches from chin	2 points
Knee 12 inches from chin	1 point

7. Arm Raise.   Sitting or standing, extend your arms out to the sides so that they are parallel to the floor. With your shoulders flat (check them in a mirror, or ask your fitness buddy to check them), raise your arms above your head until your hands touch. Score yourself as follows:

Elbows straight	5 points
Elbows slightly bent	4 points
Elbows sharply bent	3 points
Elbows sharply bent, hands cannot touch	2 points
Elbows sharply bent, hands can touch ears	1 point

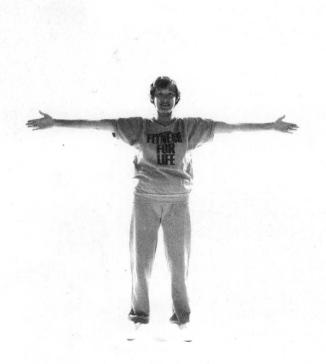

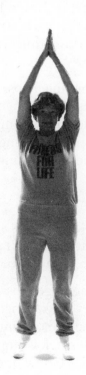

8. Leg Raise.   (This is not for bad backs.) Lying on your back (supine) on a carpet or firm bed, place your hands behind your head. Keep your legs together and lift them a few inches; try to keep your knees as straight as you can. H-o-l-d as long as possible. Time yourself, or have someone time you. Then rate yourself.

More than 10 seconds   5 points
6 to 9 seconds   4 points
2 to 5 seconds   3 points
0 to 1 second   2 points
Barely raised   1 point

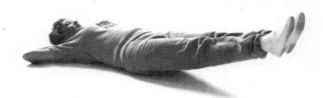

9. Sit-up.   Still supine, place your hands behind your head. Anchor your feet by either hooking them under a heavy piece of furniture (such as a chair) or having someone gently sit on them. Before you begin, draw your legs up so that your knees are bent. Now pull your trunk up to the sitting or near sitting position. Score yourself as follows:

Full sitting position   5 points
3/4 sitting position   4 points
1/2 sitting position   3 points
1/4 sitting position   2 points
Barely up   1 point

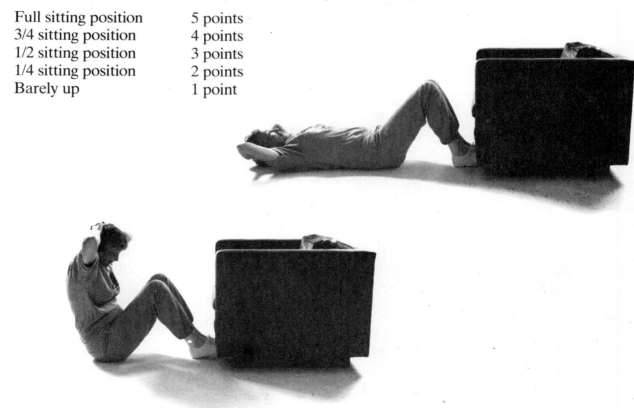

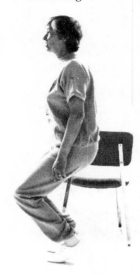

10. Knee Bend.   Stand alongside the back of a chair, preferably with someone sitting in the chair. Keeping your back straight, lower yourself by bending your knees. Do *not* try to go all the way down—you don't want to pull a muscle or tendon. Count the number of times you can raise yourself.

5 bends and raises	5 points
4 bends and raises	4 points
3 bends and raises	3 points
2 bends and raises	2 points
1 bend and raise	1 point

11. Modified Push-up.   This should be done on the floor on a rug, towel, or mat. Get down on your hands and knees. Distribute your weight so that your lower body is supported by your bent knees and your upper body is supported by your straightened arms. Rest on your hands, with your fingers pointing forward. Keeping your back straight, lower your chest to the floor. Just as you touch, push yourself up to the starting position. Count the maximum number you can do for your score.

10 push-ups	5 points
7 to 9 push-ups	4 points
4 to 6 push-ups	3 points
1 to 3 push-ups	2 points
Barely up	1 point

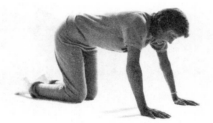
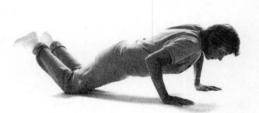

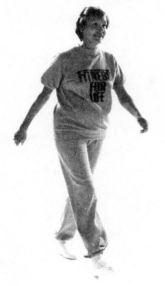

12. Walking.   Walk briskly (outside if weather permits) and measure the length of time it takes for you to get winded. Score yourself as follows:

16 to 20 minutes	5 points
11 to 15 minutes	4 points
6 to 10 minutes	3 points
1 to 5 minutes	2 points
Below 1 minute	1 point

13. Arm Pinch.   Raise one arm so that the thumb and fingers of the other hand can grab the flesh at the back of your upper arm. Pinch lightly and keep the gap between fingers and thumb as you move them away. Measure that gap. Here's how to rate what you measure.

Less than 1/2 inch	5 points
1/2 inch to 1 inch	4 points
1 inch to 1 1/2 inches	3 points
1 1/2 inches to 2 inches	2 points
2 inches to 2 1/2 inches	1 point

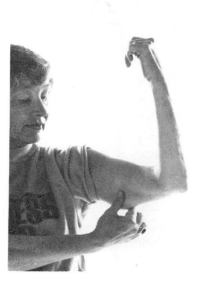
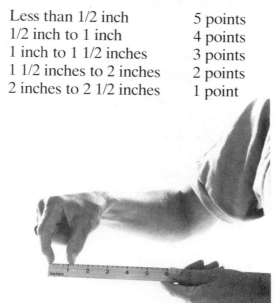

14. Waist Pinch.   With your abdominal muscles relaxed, gently pinch some of the flesh at your waistline. Measure the gap between your thumb and fingers after you move them away from your waist. Rate yourself.

Less than 1 inch	5 points
1 to 2 inches	4 points
2 to 3 inches	3 points
3 to 4 inches	2 points
4 to 5 inches	1 point

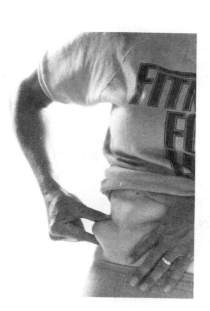
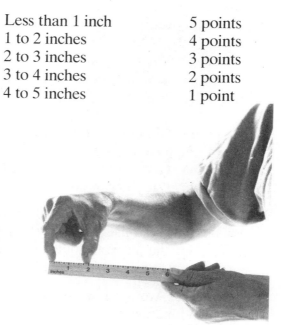

Scoring Yourself

Tests 1 through 7 measured the flexibility of various parts of your body—trunk, hips, knees, and shoulders. (35 points)
Tests 8 through 11 measured strength. (20 points)
Test 12 measured total body endurance. (5 points)
Tests 13 and 14 measured body fat. (10 points)
The total possible points you could have accumulated was 70, distributed this way.

1.	Trunk Stretch	5 points possible
2.	Hip Bend	5 points possible
3.	Toe Touch	5 points possible
4.	Leg Kick	5 points possible
5.	Side Kick	5 points possible
6.	Knee Squeeze	5 points possible
7.	Arm Raise	5 points possible
8.	Leg Raise	5 points possible
9.	Sit-up	5 points possible
10.	Knee Bend	5 points possible
11.	Modified Push-up	5 points possible
12.	Walking	5 points possible
13.	Arm Pinch	5 points possible
14.	Waist Pinch	5 points possible

Total: 70 points possible

Here's how to calculate your Functional Fitness Self-Assessment score. For an overall measure of your total body fitness, simply add up the scores of the 14 tests. As you can see from the chart above, a perfect score would be 70 points, a dreadful score 0 points. Most likely, your score is somewhere in between. Here's a guide to help you assess your fitness.

0 to 14 points: Minimum Fitness Level. You have been sitting around doing nothing for too long. Your body is stiff, weak, possibly fat, and lacks stamina. That's not an insult; it's an indication of how far you have to go to be fit. But you can do it!

15 to 28 points: Poor Fitness Level. You are at better than minimum fitness, but you may have a long way to go to get to optimum fitness level for functioning the way you would like. You will have to work, but if you take it slowly, you can achieve excellent fitness.

29 to 42 points: Average Fitness Level. You are at about average fitness. You still can function better, so start a fitness program and stick to it. If

you would like to get into a sports program, you first need to raise your fitness level.

43 to 56 points: Very Good Fitness Level. You are in pretty good shape and can start thinking about taking part in the sports you love. And you probably look terrific. But to do well in any sport, and to look even better, you need to raise the level of your fitness, so start your program now.

57 to 70 points: Excellent Fitness Level. You are ready to start planning a sports program that you can regularly participate in in order to hold the keen edge of physical fitness, to stay as healthy as you can. (But see below before you leap into the water or run onto the tennis court.)

Analyzing Your Score

This Functional Fitness Self-Assessment was positioned to meet the expected level of intensity of persons like you who have not exercised much in years. Although you are not an athlete, you are capable of using one or more exercises to raise the level of your body's fitness in order to be able to function in the lifestyle you choose.

In the unlikely event that you did make a perfect score, you may be ready to start training for some sports, if this is one of your goals. (See chapters 13 and 16.) But before you start, please note the word *ready.* If your score *is* perfect and sports is your goal, you are still not ready for competitive athletics, but you *may* be ready to start working out to get there. (Of course, sports is just one goal you may choose as part of the lifestyle you're working toward.) A perfect score on this self-assessment merely indicates a high level of fitness.

More likely, however, you've found that you need work in one or more of the areas tested. Your score in each area tells you how much work you need.

For instance, low scores on tests 1 through 7 tell you that your body's flexibility could be improved and that you should be doing exercises to improve flexibility. Which areas of the body you want to improve depends on the kind of activities in your life you want to be better at. That's where you build your wants into the design of your fitness program, especially through the exercises in chapter 5.

Likewise, low scores on tests 8 through 11 indicate a need to improve your strength. Just which muscles need strengthening depends on the functions you wish them to do. For instance, if you like to walk and want to walk more, you should strengthen your leg and foot muscles. If you want to play tennis, you also need to strengthen your hand and arm muscles. For specific exercises, see chapter 6.

If you find yourself winded easily and quickly and you thus scored low on test 12, you know that if you want to do more, you will have to work on increasing your stamina—your ability to endure in physical activity, which is best characterized by windedness. Running out of wind easily indicates you have little stamina; being able to breath easily even when expending physical effort over a period of time indicates that your stamina is adequate to the functions you wish to perform, be they daily functions or tennis. Chapter 6 instructs you on improving your stamina.

The fourth component of fitness is dealt with in chapter 7. You actually don't need a test to tell you how much "leaning" you have to do. You probably already know that. You can tell by looking at yourself nude in a full-length mirror. But the Arm Pinch and Waist Pinch tests provide objective measures of your body fat.

If you have been diligent about taking this Functional Fitness Self-Assessment and will spend a few minutes analyzing the results, you can design a program that will go a long way toward getting you to the level of fitness that will make the rest of your life more fun and more healthy. This is true at every level of activity, whether you choose that level or are bound to it by circumstances.

4 Cardiovascular Fitness

One of the primary benefits of fitness is a healthy heart and healthy blood vessels.

Even doctors who disagree on other benefits of fitness agree on this one. So you should heed the advice that the health of your cardiovascular system gets a bit better with every increment of fitness your body gains through exercise.

Your heart is a muscle. Like every other muscle in your body, it remains strong and durable with use. It weakens and withers with disuse. Like other muscles, your heart is an able servant; it will adjust itself in response to the demands you put upon it. Physical activity, through exercise or sports, is the way to make such demands. Inactivity, or failure to make demands, is the way to weaken your heart so that you fatigue easily and cannot function anywhere near the level at which you used to function or would like to function, or both.

"When I was in medical school," says Dr. Kenneth H. Cooper, director of the Aerobic Center in Dallas, Texas, "we were taught that a man past forty years of age shouldn't even jog, that it was dangerous and that he could have a heart attack. Now we have men past forty years of age approaching the four-minute mile. So, obviously there have been some major changes in our ideas and concepts in the last thirty years about what the older person can do."

The "Athletic Heart" Myth

Another misconception that has fallen behind medical progress is that of the "athletic heart." There is no such thing. The misconception was based on the false assumption that to do more work, the heart had to fill up with increased amounts of blood. This would mean it had to increase its capacity—in essence, that it had to dilate. Technically, this would force the large lower chambers, the ventricles, to balloon, thus thinning their walls and risking rupture. Medical scientists have shown

Regularly performed exercise may have a beneficial effect on the myocardial blood supply and may also protect against some of the risk factors that play major roles in the development of atherosclerosis . . . by far the major cause of disability and death in our aging population.
—John O. Holloszy, M.D., Washington University School of Medicine

that to increase its output during exercise, the heart doesn't need to *overfill;* rather, it more efficiently *empties* with each beat. As a matter of measure, athletes' hearts are within the range of normal size, though they may tend to be at the larger end of that range. In no case are the walls of the heart made thinner by exercise; thin heart walls are caused by disease unrelated to exercise.

Besides making the heart more efficient as a muscle, exercise also stimulates the blood vessels of the heart to enlarge so as to increase their ability to supply blood to meet the heart's increased demands. Furthermore, exercise also increases the flow of blood through the arteries and veins of the rest of your body. This helps prevent them from becoming clogged and helps stave off both heart attack and stroke. Research indicates that regular sessions of moderate exercise, followed by regular rest periods, are better for the arteries than constant, heavy exercising.

Research also indicates that exercise helps the heart by increasing levels of high-density lipoprotein (HDL). These complexes of protein and fat may protect against atherosclerosis, which is the major cause of heart attack in the Western world. HDL is the "good guy" in the fight against atherosclerosis, that disease in which the arteries of the heart gradually become clogged with deposits of fat and cholesterol. This suggests that exercise-induced HDL levels may help reverse the stopping up of these coronary arteries and thus help prevent heart attack.

Increased HDL levels were also involved in a landmark British study of nearly eighteen-thousand civil service workers that showed that middle-aged men (ages forty to sixty-five) who exercised regularly experienced half the incidence of coronary heart disease of fellow workers who did not exercise regularly. This was due to increased HDL levels, the increased efficiency of their hearts, and increased blood flow, said the researchers at the London School of Hygiene and Tropical Medicine in 1980. Their results were confirmed by a Los Angeles study that was reported in 1983. The eight-year study involved nearly three-thousand policemen and firemen between the ages of thirty-five and fifty-five. It showed that those men who exercised regularly had half the heart attack rate of similar men who did not exercise regularly. And a study at Penn State, also reported in 1983, showed that middle-aged *women* are similarly protected from heart disease by regular exercise.

Exercise also aids the heart by helping burn off extra calories, helping to keep the body slim, thus reducing the sedentary work load of the heart. Creeping obesity is a problem for most people in developed nations. It comes with the body's decreased need for calories with aging, with easily available food, and with the comfortable living circumstances of our modern mechanized society.

According to the National Center for Health Statistics, by the time most adults reach middle age, they find that they have gained twenty-five or thirty pounds or more and that they are eating more and exercising less than when they were young adults. And, unless they have been exercising regularly and consistently, their heart and blood vessels are in some stage of disease. Exercise can help reverse that condition— can improve the health of heart and blood vessels.

Activity Versus Rest

But you have to remember that these beneficial effects of exercise are *not permanent.* They come only after a great deal of exercising. They diminish when exercise, once begun, is cut back. They disappear when exercising stops.

For most people who are middle-aged and older, this concept of the benefits of physical activity runs contrary to some of the concepts of the benefits of rest upon the body. Medical scientists have shown that rest—by itself—is not always helpful; after a period of exercise, though, it is helpful.

The myth of the benefits of rest stems in part from the appreciation of the luxury of rest that our immigrant, physically laboring forebears passed on to us. The other part of the myth comes from the Rate of Living theory of the Roaring Twenties. The chief advocate of this theory was Dr. R. Pearl, who entreated all to save energy in youth in order to increase life span. According to this theory, the greater the rate of energy expenditure the shorter the life span. In other words, the myth proposed—and many people believed it—that rigorous physical activity wore you out.

"On the contrary," wrote Dr. John O. Holloszy, of the Department of Preventive Medicine at Washington University School of Medicine, St. Louis. "In contrast to machines that wear out more rapidly the more they are used, the tissues and organs of vertebrates develop an adaptive increase in functional capacity in response to increased use, which runs counter to the changes that occur with age. . . . A good example of the role of exercise in increasing and maintaining functional capacity is the adaptive response of the cardiovascular system."

He pointed out that exercise not only increases the efficiency of the heart and arteries but also increases the efficiency and capacity of the lungs by forcing them to adapt to working harder. This means that the lungs increase their ability to oxygenate, or freshen, blood.

For all the reasons that exercise helps the healthy heart, it also helps the heart that has recovered from an attack—otherwise known as myocardial infarct or MI. Cardiologists now insist that persons who have survived an MI almost immediately get on an exercise-therapy program in the hospital. It usually begins with passive exercises, in which arms and legs and neck are manipulated by a nurse or therapist to help restore flexibility. This progresses to in-bed exercises, sitting exercises, and walking exercises, which are continued and extended when the patient returns home.

Once the heart attack survivor is medically stable, the physician prescribes an exercise recovery program that is based on the results of a battery of tests, including the stress test. Dr. Samuel Fox, director of the Cardiology Exercise Program at Georgetown University Hospital, Washington, D.C., found that exercise not only prevents heart attack but also produces a 25 percent improvement in function. A Louisiana study showed that most cardiac patients can exercise at normal levels three months after discharge. "Normal" was defined as thirty to sixty minutes of exercise three to five days a week.

The Stress Test

Again, a heart patient should only go on an exercise plan that has been tailored for him or her and is heavily responsive to the results of a stress test, which measures the output potential of the heart under conditions of specific amounts of physical stress that the body has to overcome. Specifically, the doctor will be measuring *cardiac output,* which is technically derived by multiplying stroke volume (the volume of blood the heart pumps with each beat) by heart rate—both of which are limiting factors expended during an exercise test.

Analysis of the wave drawn as a graph on the strip of ECG paper during the stress test tells the doctor how well (or poorly) the entire heart is performing and how well specific parts of the heart are performing. The stress test produces an accurate profile of the heart and its performance with the lungs and with the rest of the body during physical effort. On the basis of these data, the doctor can determine how vigorous a fitness program can be in order to provide benefits and still be safe.

The stress test should be given not only to heart patients but to all persons over the age of forty who want to undertake a strenuous exercise program. The stress test is simply a means of giving your body a measured amount of physical stress and then measuring your body's reaction to this stress. When you take a stress test, you will note that the physical stress is accomplished either by your walking on a treadmill or pedaling a stationary cycle. The resistance, or work load, of either treadmill or cycle is adjusted at specific time intervals (often three minutes each) from light through moderate to heavy. What is light and what is heavy depends on your body's response.

Attached to your chest are one or more wire leads connected to an electrocardiograph, which measures and graphs the electrical activity of your heart. The electrocardiogram is a repetitive series of curve-spike-curve lines traced on a strip of special graph paper. The doctor will pay particular attention to the curve that follows the spike. This curve, called the S-T segment, offers a clear indication of the presence of coronary artery disease.

Some testing laboratories will increase the work load until your heart rate is at 100 percent of its predicted maximum. (That is calculated by subtracting your age from 220. Thus, if you are sixty, your maximum heart rate should be 160 beats per minute.) Other laboratories prefer to stress you to some percentage of your maximum rate, say 85 percent. Still other labs will keep increasing the work load until you are short of breath, feel fatigued, or experience some pain in the chest.

All the time you are working on the treadmill or cycle, someone, not a machine, will be monitoring your pulse and blood pressure to assure that you are not getting into trouble. Some laboratories also draw blood at various intervals during the test, and a few labs in addition monitor the air you breathe in and out. Both are done to assess how your body performs under aerobic conditions—those in which your muscles are burning oxygen from the air you breathe.

Best Heart Exercises

The best exercises for improving the condition of the heart are
- *brisk,* so as to raise the heartbeat and breathing rates
- *sustained,* so as to be performed at least fifteen to thirty minutes without any interruption
- *regular,* so as to be repeated at least three times per week

The most vigorous exercises for the heart are these
(in alphabetical order):

cross-country skiing (Nordic)

hiking (uphill)

ice hockey

jogging

jumping rope

running in place

stationary cycling

These are moderate heart exercises:

bicycling

downhill skiing (Alpine)

basketball

calisthenics

field hockey

handball

racquetball

soccer

squash

swimming

tennis (singles)

walking

These do not condition the heart much:

baseball

bowling

football

golf

softball

volleyball

5 Flexibility

Flexibility is being able to freely move your joints—not only the obvious joints such as your elbows, fingers, and toes, but also the hidden joints such as the vertebrae in your back.

Stiffness is a limited ability to move those joints.

While being female and living in a warm environment are factors associated with greater flexibility, and being male and living in a cold environment are associated with stiffness, most people regard flexibility and stiffness as directly proportional to youth and aging. We tend to think of young people as being very flexible and middle-aged and older persons as stiff. Generally, it is true that younger children are very flexible and that over the years flexibility is replaced by stiffness. But the stiffness is not necessarily a concomitant of aging. Stiffness is more likely the result of inactivity and disuse. The principle of "Use it or lose it" refers equally as well to joints as it does to muscles. In both cases, those that are not used tend to deteriorate. Muscles become weaker and joints become stiffer, and sometimes both situations occur at the same time.

This is not to suggest that you need to have the extreme total flexibility of a yogi or a contortionist, or even the flexibility in your hips of a hurdler, the flexibility in your shoulders of a racing swimmer, or the flexibility in your spine of a high diver or gymnast. But you do need enough flexibility to be active and to do the things you want to do, such as walking, shopping, keeping house, gardening, and engaging in your favorite hobbies and sports.

Flexibility Factors

Flexibility, or the range of possible motion in a joint, is naturally limited by the mechanical factors determined by the joint's design and construction. A knee bends in one direction; an elbow bends in one

In many parts of the world older individuals continue to be physically vigorous with strong muscles, strong bones, and supple bodies. One need look no farther than the 70- and 80-year-old Africans who are tribal dancers. Many changes noted in muscles and skeleton with age can definitely be prevented.
—Lawrence E. Lamb, M.D., Health Columnist

29

direction and twists clockwise and counterclockwise; a shoulder rotates.

There are other mechanical factors that limit range of motion. Two of them involve the tissue that lines the bones in a joint, the cartilage. Injury or disease can cause the cartilage to tear or break off. In osteoarthritis that lining can become very thin or even wear out. Without the cartilage to serve as a shock absorber and to offer a smooth surface over which the bones of the joint can slide, the bones actually rub against each other. In arthritis, spurs, or tiny points of bone, can form in the joint. This limits movement in two ways: as a mechanical impediment and because of the tenderness or pain involved with the slightest motion.

Most often, the factors limiting a joint's range of motion involve the soft tissue around the joint, specifically muscles, tendons, and ligaments.

Think of joints as biomechanical devices for accomplishing motion. All motion must be powered; muscles supply the power by contracting. In fact, the main reason for muscles in the skeletal system is to supply power against a lever (a bone such as an arm or a digit). The joint (such as an elbow or a knuckle) is the fulcrum (remember your high-school physics?) in any of these skeletal lever systems.

Each lever system has two opposing muscles, one for flexion and one for extension. In your upper arm, the biceps muscle flexes, or bends, your arm, while the triceps muscle extends, or straightens, your arm. If one of any pair of opposing muscles is significantly stronger than the other, the lack of balance of power will limit the range of motion of that joint. Back to the arm example: If your biceps is much stronger than your triceps, you may not be able to fully extend your arm. Persons who have had an arm in a cast often experience stiffness of that arm as a result of imbalance caused by the greater deterioration of one muscle over the other in a set during the months of disuse.

The 434 skeletal muscles in your body are connected to bones and other movable structures by tendons, which are cords made of white connective tissue that are flexible but do not contract as muscles do. Joints are lashed together on the outside by ligaments, which are bands of tough, fibrous tissue.

The knee is a unique joint because it has two ligaments that pass through it; they can cause unique difficulties as a result. The spine is unique because the spinal cord passes through its entire length. The spine is also unique in that the cartilage between its thirty-three bones, or vertebrae, comes in the form of thick pads called disks; also, its ligaments and muscles are long, with some running the entire length of the spine, from neck to buttocks.

In the spine, as at every joint, tendons and ligaments stay strong and flexible only if they are used. With disuse, they become weak and brittle and therefore easily subject to damage and injury. Tendons especially deteriorate with years of disuse. They may actually become so brittle that they can break. This typically occurs in a leg or arm when a person who has not exercised for twenty or so years goes out and starts shoveling snow a foot thick, or suddenly starts a vigorous program of physical fitness without planning and without warming-up sessions.

The combination of weak muscles, weak tendons, and weak ligaments makes it difficult to do even ordinary, everyday activities.

Take standing up from a chair. Many sedentary older persons are so stiff that they have to lift themselves by pushing their hands on the armrests.

Consider walking up stairs. Some persons feel so stiff that they need to pull themselves up by their hands, using the banister.

In both instances, arms are brought in to assist because hip joints and thigh muscles are so out of shape and so weak that they cannot raise the weight of the body.

Besides being weak, unused muscles also are not very flexible and are shortened. These effects of disuse contribute to restricted range of motion and to feelings of stiffness in hip, back, knee, and other joints. Also like unused tendons, unused muscles can rupture under stress and produce a painful, debilitating, and potentially dangerous situation.

The Role of Exercise

As you can see, lack of exercise sets up the groundwork for physical disaster. More positively, regular exercise contributes to flexibility, maintains range of motion (or even improves it), allows you to function as you wish, and helps prevent stiffness and injuries.

Exercise can also help minimize, even relieve, the stiffness and pain of arthritis. It does this by preventing the joints from "freezing" in one position and by strengthening the muscles, tendons, and ligaments so that the joints have stability and support. In short, exercise can break the usual arthritic cycle of pain-disuse-weakness-pain. (But check with your doctor first.)

The best exercises for improving flexibility are gentle cycling, walking, calisthenics, dance, and yoga—as long as what you do involves motion of the joints and some stretching. Be careful here. The worst thing to do is start an active stretching program after you have done nothing physical for many years. Remember, your flexibility was not lost suddenly, so you will not regain it suddenly or even in a week. If you try, you may tear a tendon or a muscle or dislocate a joint. But if you do follow a program that starts very gently to restore motion and to lengthen slightly tendons and muscles, you can succeed.

Another aid to flexibility is warmth. That means two things. One is that you should exercise where the air is warm. If you exercise outside in the winter, make sure you are dressed warmly enough. The other is that you spend enough time warming up so that the internal temperature of your muscles and tendons is significantly raised. The best way to accomplish this if you are returning to exercise and sports after many years is simply to do the exercise or sport at a slow rate and at a low level of intensity. With time, you can increase both the rate and intensity—but only after proper slow and gentle warm-up each time.

If you are to regain a decent measure of flexibility to your body, you really need a lot of consistency and patience. And you need a sense of reality. You will never regain all the flexibility you had at twenty—somewhat because of age but mostly because of disuse. But you can regain a fair measure of it with exercise. (Be sure you warm up and cool down. See chapter 14.)

Muscle Strength and Endurance

There is a growing body of experimental evidence to show that healthy old individuals improve their functional capacities through physical conditioning much as do young people. Percentagewise their improvement is comparable to that in the young.
—Professor Herbert A. deVries, University of Southern California

When someone says, "muscles," you may think of strength and bulk (as on a weight lifter's body). That's a popular misconception. Bulk contributes little or nothing to function. It only looks good to those who judge and admire Mr. and Ms. Universe and to others who are involved in body sculpting. Actually, the three most important muscle function factors are strength, power, and endurance, the subject of this chapter.

Strength is the ability of a muscle to exert force.

Power is the ability of a muscle to apply force with speed.

Endurance is the ability of a muscle to engage in prolonged activity—either to repeat movements or to hold a load or position for a prolonged period of time.

You can see how strength, power, and endurance are connected. Both power and endurance apply a time factor to strength. In the case of power, short times are desirable. A muscle that can do a measured amount of work twice as fast as another muscle is considered twice as powerful. In the case of endurance, long times are desirable. To achieve endurance, you need muscle strength plus other bodily factors.

Power is important in athletic competition but is not important to functional fitness.

Strength

If a muscle is not strong, it cannot exert force—even a relatively weak force—for very long. A muscle's strength is based on its structure. The muscles discussed here are technically known as skeletal muscles because they are attached to the bones of the skeleton and have the purpose of making those bones (vertebrae, limbs, and digits) move. Other kinds of muscles in your body are the cardiac muscle of the heart and the smooth muscle found in the walls of internal organs and blood vessels.

Skeletal muscles are made of cells (muscle fibers) that are bound up in bundles of 150 or so. Because they appear striped under the microscope, they are called striated muscles. These muscle fibers are generally categorized as fast-twitch or slow-twitch fibers.

Everyone has a personal proportion of fast-twitch and slow-twitch fibers in his or her muscles. These highly individualistic ratios help determine each person's physical capabilities. For example, among athletes, sprinters have a predominance of fast-twitch fibers, while long-distance runners have a predominance of slow-twitch fibers. Exercise and training cannot change the ratio of fast to slow; rather, fast-twitch and slow-twitch fibers increase their ability to do more work in response to the kind of exercise performed.

No matter the kind of muscle fiber, as it fatigues, it becomes irritated and then is unable to respond well to commands. What makes a muscle strong is the presence of other muscle fibers that are well developed and able to take over the task of fatigued muscle fibers. In a weak muscle, there is no such easy alternating of fibers that work and fibers that rest because just about all the fibers are underdeveloped from lack of exercise.

It is important to state here that in order to develop your muscles (and their fibers), you don't need to train like an Olympic athlete. You need only exercise enough to support the kind of physical activities that maintain your lifestyle. That means that in order for you to achieve functional fitness, your muscles have to be strong enough to serve you and have the endurance necessary for maintaining whatever service you require for as long as you wish.

Size and strength are not the same. Big muscles are not necessarily strong muscles—and vice versa. Sure, those gigantic muscles of body builders look super strong. In reality they can perform only at a fraction of the strength of muscles that have been trained for performance rather than looks. Swimmers, runners, and baseball players are examples of athletes with muscles that are strong in performance but weak in macho looks. So it is not the bulk of a muscle that determines its ability to perform but its strength, power, and endurance.

Endurance

Strength is an internal factor, one that resides in the muscle itself. Endurance relies on strength plus other factors that involve the rest of the body:

- A good blood supply is necessary to bring fuel (in the form of oxygen and sugar) and to take away the waste products of muscular action (carbon dioxide, water, and lactic acid). Blood is pumped by the heart, which is made more efficient in its work by exercise, which also helps keep arteries and veins open.

- Carbohydrates in food that you eat and digest provide sugar. Sugar is picked up by blood passing through vessels in the small intestine. Exercise enhances the body's ability to metabolize sugar.

- The air you breathe in provides oxygen. Oxygen is picked up by blood passing through the lungs. At the same time, blood gives up its burden of carbon dioxide to the lungs for exhalation. Exercise develops the lungs so as to increase their ability to oxygenate blood. Blood depends on iron in its hemoglobin molecule to carry the oxygen; that iron comes from foods such as liver and red meats.

You have probably heard about aerobics. The word *aerobic* means "using air." The concept means that when muscles are used strenuously for long periods of time, they require oxygen from the bloodstream. Walking a mile or two fast is an example of an aerobic activity.

By contrast, muscles used strenuously for short periods of time are in *anaerobic* activity—they don't need oxygen from the bloodstream. Sprinting for fifty yards is an example of anaerobic activity.

Those who promote aerobics or aerobic exercising (especially Dr. Kenneth Cooper, director of the Aerobic Center, Dallas, who popularized the term) explain that by demanding oxygen, muscles exercised into the aerobic state enhance their ability to use even more oxygen, enhance the heart's ability to move blood (the heart is a muscle), enhance the blood's ability to deliver oxygen, and enhance the lungs' ability to move oxygen into the blood. So, if you can exercise yourself into an aerobic state, you will vastly increase your body's performance capabilities, its functional capabilities, and, of course, its endurance.

But aerobics is not for everyone. Whether or not you should, can, or want to undertake exercise at this level of intensity will depend on your physical state and on your life goals. If you are considering it, consult your physician first.

Deterioration

Lazy muscles deteriorate. So do lazy lungs, a lazy heart, and the rest of a lazy body.

It's that simple and that sad.

Many of the bodily changes that occur through the years that have been attributed to aging should instead be attributed to a lazy body. Laziness, not years, causes a major retreat in strength and endurance. According to Dr. Herbert A. deVries, of the University of Southern

California, the aging process per se causes but a few percentage points of falloff in muscle strength, endurance, cardiac output, and pulmonary performance. That leaves overindulgent diet and lack of physical activity as the two greatest factors in causing the so-called effects of aging on muscle strength, endurance, heart, and lungs.

The only important deterioration of fitness that is truly due to age seems to occur in the blood vessels, with hardening and narrowing that impairs blood flow, especially in the arteries. But even this aging effect in many persons often can be significantly reversed by proper diet and exercise.

A muscle shrinks and weakens with disuse (*atrophy* is the medical word) as its fibers shrink and weaken; the underused muscle doesn't lose fibers, as you might think. This weakening and shrinking are so gradual and sometimes so imperceptible that you probably won't even notice the loss until you call upon the muscle to perform. Then the pain and shortness of breath you will experience will probably shock you into reality.

Training

Exercises to build strength and stamina need to be done according to three general principles:

1. *Load.* To improve a muscle's strength and/or endurance, you have to press it beyond its normal, everyday load of work. A muscle will respond only to challenge. Give it a light load and it will do nothing to increase its strength. But give it a maximum load and it will strengthen its fibers and be ready for that new load the next time. But if there is no next time, it will atrophy back to its weakened previous condition.

    Athletes use this principle in their training. Swimmers train at double their competition distances so that when they do compete, they can literally sail down the lanes. Baseball players use weighted bats so that when they step up to the plate with a regulation bat, it feels light. Football quarterbacks use weights to develop their legs and lower body muscles so that they can have the power to break tackles when they are running down the field with the ball. You are probably not interested in competitive sports, but your ability to use your arms, or your legs, and to use them for longer periods of time than before can be improved by following this principle.

2. *Alternate Days.* Don't do strength and endurance exercises every day. Rather, do them on alternate days so that one day you exercise hard and the next day you exercise easy. This gives the muscles a chance to catch up and to build up their fibers in

order to meet the new challenge. Think of it this way: Each new stress on a muscle causes minor injuries to some of its fibers. They need time to repair; that's the easy day.

There are two other technical reasons. One is that glycogen, a starch that in essence is muscle fuel, must be replenished. The other reason is that potassium, used by the muscle to control heat, is depleted and needs to be replenished.

3. *Specificity.* A muscle will respond in a specific way to the load. It will respond exactly to the angle, speed, and challenge of the load, and not to any other. For example, if you walk briskly up hills, the muscles of your legs will strengthen and increase their endurance so that any fatigue and pain you experienced at the beginning of such exercising will disappear. Better yet, when you then walk at a strolling pace on a level sidewalk, it will seem effortless. But your swimming will not have been strengthened, nor will your tennis game have been improved.

Exercising for Strength

Exercises that strengthen your muscles are those that you do against force. The more your muscle contracts against a force, the more strength it can develop. Strengthening exercises are classified as *isometric, isotonic, isokinetic,* and *active.* Here are the differences.

- *Isometric exercises* made Charles Atlas rich and famous. These are the kinds of exercises that cause muscles to contract without their moving any limbs or joints. For instance, as you sit reading this book, your elbows are probably resting on the arms of a chair or on your lap. If you press down hard on your elbows so as to put a lot of weight on them, you will be contracting muscles in your abdomen, upper arms, and sides. Nothing need move in this exercise. Yet, you are contracting those muscles against a force. Similarly, if you raise your arm and contract your biceps for thirty seconds, then rest, then contract again, and so on, you will be strengthening your biceps without moving your forearm—which is the biceps's job.

  Isometric exercises work. They do strengthen muscles. But they are not usually recommended because that is all they do. They do *not* help endurance because they lack movement and because they have no effect on the cardiovascular system or lungs. They even may be dangerous because they cause brief rises in blood pressure and can adversely affect heart rhythm. Thus, they are in the same category as an absolutely sedentary middle-aged person suddenly going out and shoveling a walk covered with two feet of snow.

- *Isotonic exercises* are characterized by weight lifting. Like isometrics, these exercises employ the contraction of muscle against a heavy force; unlike isometrics, isotonics move limbs or joints, or both—but not very much. The idea is to exert pressure against a maximum force for sets of ten repetitions. Unfortunately, isotonics (also called isophasics) do little to improve the cardiovascular system or the lungs and thus add nothing to your endurance. All that can be said for isotonics is that they build strength and also bulk. They are not recommended for most middle-aged or older persons.

- *Isokinetic exercises* are characterized by the new popularity of exercise machines such as those built by Nautilus or Universal Gym. They use the principle of weight as a force to make a muscle contract, but they introduce a full range of motion. Unlike weight training, which requires you to lift a weight against gravity and then allows gravity to lower the weight, in isokinetics you have to use your muscles both to lift and lower the weight. This kind of exercising not only strengthens muscles but also adds to endurance because it extends the length of time the muscles are working.

- *Active exercises* are the kind that require you to move your body and its limbs. These exercises build strength *and* endurance. At the same time, they help your heart and lungs and aid flexibility. Active exercises can be anaerobic or aerobic (see page 35).

None of these kinds of exercises is better or worse than the other kinds. Rather, each kind is good for specific purposes. However, if you had to decide on one over the others, it should be active exercises, since they accomplish more of the kinds of results you probably are striving for. In other words, active exercises are more efficient in a fitness program.

However, active exercises are not always as convenient as the others. You have to bend and twist; you have to walk, run, or swim. Isometrics are the most convenient, since they require no equipment. Isotonics are slightly less convenient, since they require simple equipment such as dumbbells, which you may have at home. Isokinetics are the least convenient, since they require sophisticated equipment that you are not likely to have at home.

Exercising for Endurance

The way you build endurance is by loading muscles, lungs, and the cardiovascular system in a progressive manner. That means that you start modestly, pushing yourself a little more at each stage, until you have achieved your goal—whether it is a specific pulse rate or blood pressure or some physical achievement such as walking a mile.

The most difficult part is getting started. But once you are well into your exercise program, you will feel wonderfully stronger and more able to do things—and for longer.

You will be able to tell how your endurance is stretching by your breathlessness. When you begin exercising, you may experience breathlessness very soon, but as you progress in your exercise program, you will note that it takes more and more to take your breath away. That's one of the best and clearest signs of endurance. Another is muscle soreness, which you will experience at the beginning of your program and then not again once your endurance has developed.

The best endurance exercises are those that require many repetitions over time, such as walking, swimming, cycling, jogging, and tennis.

As you surmise, the best exercises at every level of intensity are those that are active, aerobic, and continuous. You have to pick the specific ones that suit your physical condition and your lifestyle when you put your exercise program together.

Finally, here is a ranking of sixteen sports activities by strength and endurance benefits. The data, gathered by the President's Council on Physical Fitness and Sports, represent total points accumulated from seven physical fitness experts asked to do the rankings.

Sport	*Endurance Benefit*	*Strength Benefit*
Jogging	20	17
Swimming	20	14
Skiing, cross-country	19	15
Bicycling	18	16
Skiing, downhill	18	15
Handball and squash	18	15
Skating, ice and roller	17	15
Basketball	17	15
Tennis	16	14
Walking	14	11
Calisthenics	13	16
Golf	8	9
Softball	8	7
Bowling	5	5

7 Leanness

Exercise does cause a decrease of body weight without alterations in the diet. The fact that athletes engaged in endurance sports are thin is well-established. Longitudinal observations show that skinfolds decrease during training periods without any restriction in dietary intake.
—Per Bjorntorp, M.D., University of Göteborg, Sweden

You have seen the concept of the ideal figure change perhaps more than once. Back at the beginning of the twentieth century, heavy was regarded as healthy because slim was akin to consumptive, or tubercular. Grandparents loved to pinch the cheeks of fat babies and worried about babies who were not chubby. Beautiful women were buxom or "full-figured." Healthy men were rotund.

Today, thanks to medical research, we know that slim is not only "in" but also healthy. So if you are not now slim, you should think of slim as a fitness goal.

And exercise can help you.

In addition to helping to keep you healthy enough, strong enough, and flexible enough to do what you want to do, exercise will *help* you reverse the sagging and softness of your body—a body that may have been left behind by years of inactivity or underactivity.

Notice the word *help*. That's what exercise can do if you want to slim down. But exercise will not do it alone.

To effectively lose weight (and fat), you need to combine exercise with a cutback of calories on a well-rounded diet. The roles of exercise are to tighten skin loosened as fat leaves and to harden the muscles below the skin, which have not had much chance in quite a while to show their form.

Slimming Your Body

To slim your body, you have to understand and follow the following six principles, perform the kind of exercises that produce leanness, and be realistic in your goals.

1. Exercise Firms You Up

The first principle is that a body does not get soft and flabby because of aging or because of a physical handicap. Rather, soft-and-

41

flabby is a sign of unfitness. There are men and women of all ages and with various kinds of handicaps who have lean, firm bodies. But the firmness and leanness didn't just happen; these conditions required exercise. Bodies remain firm and lean only with regular exercise.

What was said earlier about fitness being a temporary condition is also true of leanness. Like fitness, leanness is dependent on exercise. Leanness stays only with exercise; it leaves, letting fat and flab too quickly take its place, when exercise is stopped.

Leanness and fitness creep in; flab and poor shape gallop in.

2. There Are No Spot-reducing Exercises

The second principle is that you can firm up portions of all of your body, but you have little control over specific fat deposits. In plainer language, this means that you cannot spot-reduce, no matter what the health club hucksters advertise.

Where fat accumulated on your body and in what concentrations were initially determined as you entered adolescence. And there is a sex difference. Men tend to deposit excess fat behind the abdominal wall (often producing a "beer belly") as well as at other sites above the navel. Women tend to deposit fat below the navel, especially on hips, buttocks, and thighs.

Of course, female breasts are largely rounded deposits of fat. Still, women are not all created equal. They do not universally put on and take off fat from their breasts as they gain and lose weight. Some women do; some do not.

Other sites of extra fat deposition on your body—such as under the chin and at the back of the upper arms—are determined by genetics, over which you have no influence. So while you can expect dieting to reduce your *total* body fat, you cannot diet to reduce fat at any *specific* place on your body while sparing other places. It just doesn't work that way. Frustrating though the situation may be to you, the control of where you lose fat as you lose weight lies in the genes you inherited from your parents. There is nothing you can do about that— even in the last years of the twentieth century.

3. Exercise Flattens the Tummy

Another principle: On only two areas of the body, both broad surfaces, can you expect exercise to help reduce fat. These are on the trunk, under the skin of the upper back and the abdomen. Some people have fatty backs, but there are probably lots more with protruding tummies (or perhaps it is that tummies are more visible).

The best exercises for tightening your tummy are sit-ups, head curls, leg raises, walking, and jogging—in short, every activity that uses abdominal muscles. And the more repetitions, the better, as explained on the following page.

It's important to inject a caveat here. These exercises will reduce the fat *in front of* the abdominal muscles. But they will do nothing for the fat *behind* the muscles. That fat accumulates on the omentum, which is the tissue that holds the internal organs together. The only way you can lose such inner fat is to reduce your total caloric intake. Another way to say this is, You won't lose your potbelly by exercise; you have to go on a diet and reduce the fat all over your body!

4. Repetitive Exercises Are the Best

The basic principle in exercising for slimming is repetition. The *more often* and the *more constantly* you exercise your abdominal muscles, the more fat you can remove and keep away from the space between those muscles and the skin above them.

More often means the number of times you do head curls (or any other exercise) at a time. The more repetitions the better. Of course, you have to start doing but a few and build up to doing many over a reasonable period of time. Otherwise you will produce soreness and other problems for yourself.

More constantly means the frequency that you repeat your abdominal exercise program. Thus every other day is better for slimming than every third day, and every day is better than every other day.

There is little difference between static and dynamic exercises in effectiveness in slimming. This means that isometric, isotonic, isokinetic, and active exercises all work, as do sports. The goal of slimming does not require that you improve your cardiovascular capacity, as endurance does. It does require that you do the same exercise every day, day in and day out, and for the number of repetitions that do the job.

Sound boring?

A lot of people think so, judging from their potbellies. There is no denying the fact that repetitive exercises such as morning calisthenics are boring. OK, that's a given. If you are determined, that won't matter; you'll put on some music or exercise with your spouse or a buddy in order to pass the time more interestingly. Those who are not determined will use it as an excuse to accomplish nothing. The choice is yours, as it always is.

5. Exercise Dulls Appetite

Another principle of slimming is that exercise helps by curbing appetite.

It is a physiological fact that exercising releases stored energy into the blood in the form of carbohydrates, fat globules, and ketone bodies. In addition to providing energy to the muscles, these nutrients also have the effect of holding appetite down. Two of these (carbohydrates and fats) are the same nutrients that enter the bloodstream from your small intestine after you eat. When these nutrients get into the blood, you have a feeling of being satiated. But the appestat, which controls your appetite, doesn't know the source of those chemicals; it just knows they are in the blood. Since the blood is rich in these nutrients, it reasons, why stimulate appetite?

Exercise has another benefit toward slimming. It boosts the metabolism so that energy stores of the body are burned not only during the duration of the exercise but also for at least six hours thereafter. That means that you burn extra calories, above and beyond what you expend by physical effort and for hours after your exercise session has ended.

According to Dr. Herbert A. deVries of the University of Southern California, this effect of exercise can result in a weight loss of four to five pounds a year.

6. Dieting Is the Best Way to Lose Weight

This leads to another principle: Dieting, not exercise, is the best way to lose weight. This is because you lose weight as a result of using (burning) more calories than you eat. It's strictly a deficit question. You want your body to be in caloric deficit. Exercise uses more calories than sitting around does. But you cannot create as much of a caloric deficit with exercise as you can with dieting.

Certainly, athletes—amateur and professional alike—have muscular bodies with little fat. But they exercise for several hours every day. You are not at all likely to be willing (or able) to devote that kind of time and energy to working out. Exercise should be a means of achieving and maintaining functional fitness, being able to do what you want to do in life. Exercise should not be an all-consuming activity of its own. Such dedication and compulsion are appropriate for athletes, not for you.

Here are the numbers that make the case.

To lose a pound, you need to burn up 3,500 more calories than you eat. The easiest, most consistent way to achieve a caloric deficit of 3,500 is to eat that many fewer calories. So if you want to lose a pound a week, you simply lower your daily caloric intake by 500 calories (500 × 7 = 3,500). That means that if you are used to eating 2,500 calories a day, you can lose a pound a week by eating only 2,000 calories a day (2,500 − 500 = 2,000).

Incidentally, this arithmetic applies even over a longer span of time. These hard numbers don't care about your time frame, only that the energy deficit exists. So you could lose a pound over two weeks by eating 3,500 calories less in *two* weeks instead of one. That comes to 250 fewer calories a day, of course, rather than 500.

To lose a pound a week by exercise alone, you have to do any of the following very strenuous activities every day for seven days: walk briskly for two and a half hours (at 2.3 mph), swim the crawl for an hour and fifteen minutes (at 1 mph), climb stairs for an hour (at a rate of three flights a minute, up and down), ski cross-country for fifty-six minutes (at the rate of 3 mph), cycle for 2.6 hours (at 5.5 mph), jog thirty-six minutes (at 5.5 mph).

A bit impractical for most of us!

The very best way to slim is to combine repetitive exercising *with* a reduction in calories. That combination gives you a multiplying effect. Dr. Frank Konishi of Southern Illinois University has devised a wonderful plan for achieving this. For instance, if you walked thirty minutes a day and cut back 400 calories a day by dieting, you could lose five pounds in twenty-seven days. Or, if you instead swam for thirty minutes a day and cut back the same 400 calories from food, you would lose five pounds in twenty-three days. Once you are in good physical condition, you'll be able to achieve this.

Lowering your caloric intake and keeping it lowered is very difficult. But it can be done. To be successful at dieting, you need to be motivated, and you need to completely and permanently change your eating habits. This means developing new habits to replace the old ones. Some people can accomplish this on their own, but most successful dieters join a group of some kind. Few people, if any, ever lose weight and keep it off on those fad diets that come along every few months.

Make Sure Your Diet Is Balanced

It is not good enough to merely cut calories if you want to lose weight. You have to also be sure that the foods you eat on that reduced-calories diet provide you with the nutrition you require. This means that you must receive *all* essential nutrients: proteins, carbohydrates, fats, vitamins, and minerals. Here is a quick guide.

Proteins

Considered the most important of the nutrients, since it provides the raw material for building tissues in the body, protein is often misunderstood. Abundant in such animal foods as meat, milk, and eggs, it also is found in nuts, cereals, and whole-grain products. Quality, rather than abundance, should be your main concern. Protein from animal sources is generally of higher quality than is protein from plants. But you can eat vegetarian and still get high-quality protein providing you combine the protein sources. For instance, peanut butter by itself does not provide high-quality protein. But add wheat protein to peanut protein and you can give the body a high-quality combination protein. That's why a peanut butter and jelly sandwich may give you as much high-quality protein as a meat sandwich does. No matter the quality, protein yields 4 calories per gram. Protein contributes to a feeling of satiation that lasts for an hour or two after you eat. According to the National Academy of Sciences–National Research Council, the Recommended Dietary Allowance of protein is 56 grams daily if you are a man, and 44 grams if you are a woman. To give you some idea of what this means in food terms, a cup of cottage cheese contains about 30 grams of protein; two eggs, 12 grams; a 3-oz. fillet of ocean perch, 16 grams; a 3-oz. hamburger patty, 23 grams; 3 oz. of turkey meat, 26 grams; a cup of spaghetti and meatballs, 19 grams; a cup of oatmeal, 5 grams; a cup of peanuts, 37 grams.

Carbohydrates

Carbohydrates are available to the body as fuel either as sugar or starch. Sugars such as glucose, sucrose, fructose, mannose, and lactose are known as "simple" carbohydrates and are found in fruits, jams, jellies, honey, milk, and milk products. Starches, or "complex" carbohydrates, are found in breads, pasta, cereals, and vegetables and when digested are converted into the simple sugar, glucose. Complex carbohydrates contribute to satiation after you eat, while sugars make you feel fine right away but hungry in an hour. During fasting and severe dieting, the body can even make sugar from body protein and body fats. Carbohydrates yield 4 calories per gram. You need at least 60 grams of carbohydrate a day. Carbohydrate-rich foods are also a good source of vitamins, minerals, and dietary fiber. To give you some idea of what this means in food terms, a cup of ice cream contains 28 grams of carbohydrate; a raw apple, about 25 grams; a cup of orange juice, 26 grams; a bagel, 30 grams; a cup of oatmeal, 23 grams; a segment of pizza, 22 grams; a brownie, 13 grams; a tablespoon of honey, 17 grams; a baked potato, 33 grams.

Fats

Animal fat (such as lard and butter) and vegetable oils and margarine contain the same amounts of calories, 9 per gram. However, animal fats are largely of the saturated kind and have a direct effect on increasing the cholesterol content of your blood. Most plant oils (such as corn and safflower oils) are polyunsaturated and help lower blood cholesterol levels and thus are better for your heart and arteries. Fats are an important part of cell walls in the tissues of your body and also are necessary to keep your skin from drying out. Fat is the major form of energy storage in the body. Most people in our society cannot stick to diets that are much less than 25 to 30 percent fat (by calories), for two reasons. One is that fat carries so much of the flavor of food; the other is that fat provides most of the long-term satiation, the stick-to-your-ribs-for-several-hours quality of a square meal. Dietary fat also provides the body with the essential fatty acids; one-third of your daily calories should come from fat. That would be 400 calories of a diet of 1,200 calories. To give you some idea of what this means in food terms, a cup of whole milk contains 72 fat calories; a cup of ice cream, 126 fat calories; a pat of margarine, 36 fat calories; two scrambled eggs, 126 fat calories; a tablespoon of mayonnaise, 99 fat calories; a 3-oz. hamburger patty, 90 fat calories; two slices of bacon, 72 fat calories; four chocolate chip cookies, 108 fat calories; a cup of peanuts, 648 fat calories; 10 strips of french fried potatoes, 63 fat calories.

Alcohol

Alcohol also provides calories to the body. Since it is a product of fermented sugar, and thus a more concentrated form of energy, you might guess that its caloric density is greater than that of sugar. You're right—about 7 calories per gram. Alcohol is consumed more for its effects on behavior and feelings than for its limited nutritional value. If you drink, remember that moderation is necessary not only for preventing loss of control but for keeping you from gaining weight. Dieters who drink often fail to lose weight because they have failed to consider the amount of calories in their alcoholic beverages. To give you some idea, a can of beer contains 150 calories; a shot of gin, vodka, or whisky or a glass of dry wine, 100 calories each; a Manhattan, 164 calories; a martini, 140 calories; an old-fashioned, 179 calories; a highball, 166 calories.

Vitamins

If you eat a well-rounded diet of about 1,200 calories per day, you should be getting all the vitamins and minerals your body needs. But there is a good chance that you skimp here and there on the nutrient-dense foods such as breads, cereals, fruits, and vegetables and gorge on junk foods now and then. In order for your body to function properly, it is important to take in the Recommended Dietary Allowances of the fat-soluble vitamins A, D, and E and the water-soluble vitamins, C and B-complex. So take a multivitamin and mineral supplement if you go on a low-calorie diet in order to lose weight.

Minerals

Minerals are basic chemical elements that work cooperatively with the vitamins in a number of essential reactions of the body. Among the most important minerals are iron (for blood), magnesium, iodine (for thyroid), zinc, phosphorus (for bone), calcium (for bone), potassium, chlorine, copper, manganese, fluoride, chromium, selenium, and molybdenum. Most of these minerals are readily provided to the body in any balanced diet. As noted earlier, it may be wise for you to take a vitamin-mineral supplement when you go on a diet to lose weight.

Fiber

In the old days, what we now call fiber was known as roughage and bulk. No matter its name, it is a class of ingredient present in foods that are derived from plants, that is, from cereals, grains, nuts, seeds, fruits, and vegetables. There is no fiber in foods derived from animals.

Because humans cannot digest fiber (which is primarily cellulose), the components of food that contain fiber are usually separated from such foods as corn flour and wheat flour. That is why most breads, pastries, and noodles, although made of wheat flour, have no wheat fiber. Instead, you can buy separately the very ingredient of wheat that has been taken out so that flour can be pure white! It is sold as miller's bran (one of the best sources of fiber) and is available in a convenient form that can be sprinkled on all kinds of food dishes.

You can get fiber in fresh fruits and vegetables, too. Among the richest in fiber are apples, berries, dates, beans, peas, potatoes, and spinach. Bran cereal and almonds are also excellent sources of fiber.

Fiber is desirable because it adds bulk to your digested food and stimulates your digestive system to move things along. As the food moves through the digestive system, a tiny percentage of its calories is not absorbed. Also not absorbed perfectly is cholesterol, that villain of the heart.

Set Realistic Goals

When it comes to slimming, as it does in every other goal of exercise, be realistic. Don't expect to take inches and pounds off in a few days or even a few weeks. Because the excess fat on your body took years to put on, you can't expect it to come off overnight. That's OK. The idea is to start now and get things going in the right direction, at last.

Be patient with yourself. If you forget to exercise one day or go off your diet for a weekend, don't feel that you have failed. Rather, just regard it for what it was, a temporary aberration. Get back on the track and on the program better for the experience, knowing what it was that tempted you away. When that same temptation comes again, you'll be strong and ready for it.

Most of all, recognize that exercise has an important role to play in getting your body lean and tough again. But also recognize that it is not a solitary role. Don't expect exercise to do the whole job. You've got to cut back on the total number of calories you eat, too, and to work on breaking bad old habits and replacing them with newly developed good habits.

The best habit of all is fitness.

8 Relaxation

There is no conflict in prescribing physical exercise to alternate with rest. The one prepares for the other and the degree and extent of relaxation are likely to be increased after moderate exercise. . . . relaxation is the intensive form of rest.
—Edmund Jacobson, M.D., Ph.D., Originator of Progressive Relaxation

You may be surprised to find, amid text and pictures of exercises, a chapter on relaxation. You may feel that one reason you are physically so out of shape is that you have done too much relaxing for too many years.

If you think this, you are confusing being sedentary with being relaxed. They are quite different. For most of us, relaxation doesn't just happen; it needs to be made to occur. That implies that you have to know how to relax.

To achieve fitness, you have to learn not only the best ways to stress your muscles but also the best ways to relax them. Such relaxation will help you cope with the tensions and stresses of daily life, which are definitely the enemy of fitness and well-being. Relaxation will also enable the body to return needed oxygen to the tissues and remove the poisons that are produced in strenuous exercise.

Relaxation is also important to achieve peace within yourself, to allow perfect rest so that you can achieve what you have to and want to. By contrast, tension is uncomfortable and distracting. That's why so many people resort to tranquilizers, alcohol, marijuana, and other drugs. If they knew how to relax, they would not need these chemicals, and they would be far more fit and far happier than they are now.

You should find that exercise will help you relax. Fatigued muscles crave relaxation.

So will watching a movie or reading a book or listening to music help you relax. But none of these is totally relaxing because your muscles are reacting to what your mind perceives. This is also true of sleep. As you dream, just after you fall asleep and just before you awaken, your muscles react.

Scientists who have measured the electrical energy of the body find that when you think about a physical activity, read about it, view it, or dream about it, your appropriate muscles respond. Similarly, when you are emotionally aroused, your muscles tense up. Usually this tension is so slight that you don't see it or even feel it. But it is there, physically present and capable of being measured by very sensitive electrical instruments.

You have to make a time for total relaxation in your daily schedule. To achieve maximum relaxation—that is, the relaxation of as many of your 434 skeletal muscles as possible—you have to learn specific techniques such as progressive relaxation, meditation, yoga, self-hypnosis, biofeedback, or T'ai Chi Ch'uan, whichever works best for you.

Progressive Relaxation

Perhaps the greatest American researcher of relaxation is Dr. Edmund Jacobson, the Chicago physiologist and physician who wrote *You Must Relax* and *Progressive Relaxation* more than half a century ago. In 1977, he wrote, "There are reasons to believe that tension is part of the cause of many deaths each year. Possibly it kills directly or indirectly far more people than does malignancy. The prime cause of death in the United States is cardiovascular disease. In my experience progressive relaxation is of momentous importance for the prevention as well as the treatment of cardiovascular diseases."

Dr. Jacobson linked muscle tension (the opposite of relaxation) with many physical conditions and diseases, including nervousness, anxiety, insomnia, intestinal and colonic spasm, peptic ulcer, tension headaches, depression, and exhaustion. Even the stiffness and pain in joints afflicted with arthritis can be helped by relaxation.

His studies showed, by electrical measurements, that many people with these disorders do not achieve total relaxation. There is always tension in their muscles. Sometimes it can be seen in their fidgeting, leg shaking, and other nervous habits. Sometimes it can be palpated in their hard shoulder and neck muscles. Sometimes the tension can be experienced as stiffness in their joints.

He reasoned that if these patients could be taught relaxation, their disorders might get better or even go away. He tried it and claimed a high rate of success by his technique, which he called progressive relaxation.

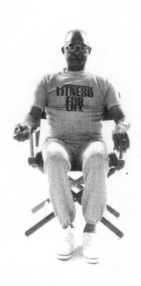

The essentials of his technique involve "muscle sense," the ability to detect tension, or contraction, in muscles. This is accomplished by voluntarily contracting one muscle group at a time and then relaxing the contraction. Try it. Rest an elbow on your chair and flex your forearm so that the hand curls upward at the wrist. The fingers and the upper arm need to be relaxed. Tighten the forearm muscle until it feels stiff. Feel the forearm muscle with the fingers of the other hand. Then suddenly let go and let the hand drop back to a resting position. Now, close your eyes and think about relaxing the forearm muscle. As you relax it, feel the forearm muscle with the fingers of the other hand. If you feel some stiffness in the muscle, you know you are not completely relaxing it; you have to work on that muscle's relaxation.

You have to develop that muscle sense in each of the muscle groups, which means both upper and lower extremities, neck, shoulders, back, chest, abdomen, and buttocks. Also, you need to "sense" the muscles in your scalp and around the eyes, the eye muscles themselves, and the jaw and facial muscles.

To relax each muscle group, you first need to contract it; then you must ease *all* contractions and tension in each muscle. You need to keep relaxing it beyond the initial feeling that it is relaxed. It has to become limp, then limper, then limper still.

This progressive relaxation is best accomplished lying supine in a quiet, semidark room. Start at your toes and work up to your scalp (which you contract by wrinkling your forehead). You should realize that mastering the art of progressive relaxation doesn't usually come quickly. It may take as long as a year to accomplish. But don't be in such a hurry. Relax!

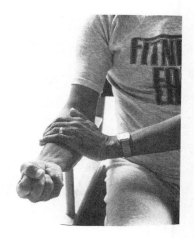

Meditation

In this generation, it has become more popular to adopt the ancient technique of relaxing called meditation. Laboratory measurements of heart rate, blood pressure, and brain waves show that it works; the measurements are lower when a person meditates.

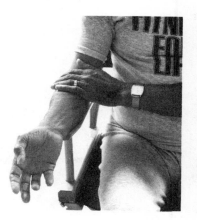

While meditation is often associated with Buddhists and Hindus, the common form in Western countries—called transcendental meditation, or TM—does not have any organized religious base. It is solely a technique for concentrating and focusing your thoughts inward. It begins by your wearing loose clothing; sitting down in a comfortable position in a quiet, darkened environment; closing your eyes; and quietly humming a single- or double-note tone, often called the *mantra,* or softly repeating a word, any word.

When you try it, you should work to concentrate on only that one sound. The principle of meditation is that this concentration will clear your mind of everything else and relax your body of its tensions.

Don't expect meditation to work instantaneously or even in five minutes. You have to set aside at least twenty minutes a day in order for meditation to accomplish the total relaxation you need. Then you will find that not only does your body feel relaxed but that also your mind feels clear—your whole self feels refreshed.

You can learn meditation on your own. In fact, you can apply these basics right now. But you will learn more details about meditation if you join a class or read a book. If you live near a city, you should be able to join a meditation class at your YMCA or YWCA or other community center, at an adult education center, or at a senior adult center.

Yoga

You should also easily be able to find a class that teaches yoga, yet another import from the East to help frenetic Westerners cope with the stress, tensions, and muscle tightness that come with everyday modern life. Yoga practitioners often meditate first. Yoga is a kind of relaxation exercise that you do after your body and mind are at ease. Like meditation, yoga requires twenty minutes, a comfortable environment, and loose clothing.

One of the best yoga teachers in North America is Lilias, an occidental who lives in Cincinnati and has often appeared on her own syndicated Public Broadcasting Service program. In her book, *Lilias, Yoga, and Your Life,* she says, "Yoga is for everyone, at any age. You can begin at any time of your life. If you are over 65 and an absolute beginner, welcome! There is no better time to start than this moment! You don't need to rush into a 5-minute headstand or a difficult pose. Just start with a weekly practice schedule and do what makes you feel comfortable and good."

Yoga, like meditation, stems from an Eastern religious practice but is taught here in its nonreligious form, hatha yoga. (Raja yoga is the religious form.)

Don't think that to do yoga you have to twist yourself into a pretzel or go into the lotus position. There are nice and easy movements that will accomplish the relaxation you seek. Here are three from Lilias.

Seated Sun Salutation
Sitting straight in a chair, bring your knees together.

Exhale, bend forward, and lay your chest on your thighs.

Clasp your hands to your elbows; then bring your arms around so they hug the knees.

Hold this position, breathing comfortably, for three to five minutes.

Inhale; then sit up straight. Keep holding your elbows.

Exhale; then lower your arms. Repeat this sit-up three times.

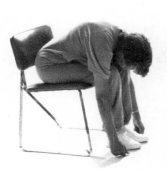 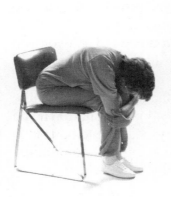 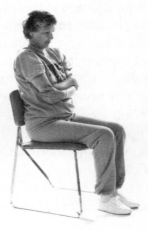 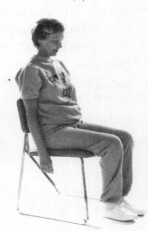

Phoenix

Lying on your abdomen, bend your elbows and place your wrists beneath your shoulders, with your fingertips pointing forward, palms down. Keep your upper arms close to your body.

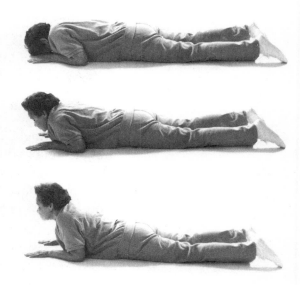

Tuck your chin close to your throat as though trying to look at your navel. Then slowly raise your forehead, nose, and chin. Raise your head up and back as far as you can. Move gently. Tighten the muscles in your buttocks and tilt your pelvis forward. At the same time, press gently down on your elbows and wrists and lift your chest even higher. Breathe comfortably. Keep your lower arms on the floor.

Slowly lower your head toward your hands, tucking in your chin toward your throat.

Repeat this three times. Move gently.

Humming Breath

Inhale smoothly, with your mouth closed. Relax your tongue and jaw. Close your eyes. Open the back of your throat as if stifling a yawn. After your lungs are completely filled, exhale by singing out the breath with a hum sound, prolonging the "m-m-m-m" as long as possible, like the hum-m-m-m of a bee. Keep the one tone as you exhale totally all the air in your lungs.

Then inhale smoothly, gently, and quietly. On exhalation, repeat the humming breath.

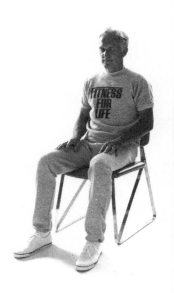

After you have done this for about three minutes, relax your hands in your lap. Imagine that you are emptying your body and mind of all tensions, negatives, and worries. Suggest to your body that it relax. Try not to doze. Your thoughts will soon quiet down, and you will be able to experience the peace that comes with each breath. Sink deeper into your inner peacefulness—into its warmth, into its light, into its calmness. Feel it expand in your chest, throat, and head. Feel it surround you. Think of a breath as a messenger that is taking positive energy to all the cells that need nourishment and healing.

Try to remain still like this for about fifteen minutes.

Self-Hypnosis

In large record stores you can buy some very good cassette tapes that will give a soft, soothing voice that lulls you into a sort of reverie that, in fact, is a form of self-hypnosis. This is not the kind of hypnosis you see on a stage, where the hypnotist makes people do funny things. Rather, this is the sort of hypnosis that makes you relax in a semisleep state from which you awaken refreshed.

While akin to meditation, self-hypnosis is different in that a voice is saying words, whether the inner voice of your mind or a voice you hear from headphones.

Biofeedback

You might call this a high-tech relaxation technique. You learn how to relax your body, emotions, and mind by using objective measurements of your brain wave activity. This is done through electrodes that are applied to your head and connected to an electronic device. You learn to produce peaceful thoughts that actually quiet the brain waves.

Similarly, you learn to relax muscles by electrodes that are applied over muscles.

You need a biofeedback machine to learn how best to quiet your waves. You can learn this from a biofeedback specialist (you'll find ads for them in the Yellow Pages under "Biofeedback Therapists"). You may want to purchase your own inexpensive home biofeedback machine so you can develop this skill to a fine point.

T'ai Chi Ch'uan

The ancient Chinese form of relaxed, gentle body movement, known popularly as T'ai Chi, is aimed at keeping the body from being tense and awkward. You can learn it from a book, but it is best learned from a teacher, a master (look in the Yellow Pages under "Karate and Other Martial Arts Instruction"). You should do this "choreography of body and mind," as it is often referred to, for about ten minutes a day. Properly done, with regulated breathing, it can ease body and mind into a state of meditation. In fact, many practitioners of T'ai Chi use the form as a preliminary to meditation.

Massage

A massage, or rubdown, is a wonderful way to relax, especially after a workout. Stick to the Swedish massage and beware of "massage parlors," which rub down more than muscles. Also, stay away from those rigorous, special kinds of massage such as rolfing, which can be injurious.

Properly applied, a massage that rubs the muscles helps relieve them of tensions and "knots" and makes you feel warm and relaxed. Of course, just lying on the massage table for a half hour or so helps. The only objective, physiological benefit that can be scientifically demonstrated from massage is removal of lactic acid—a waste product—from muscles.

Massage feels so good that you might consider it a reward for hard work at exercising.

You Must Relax!

Like exercise, relaxation must be practiced to do the maximum good. Putting it off to some indefinite future will do no good now. Relaxation is definitely *not* a waste of time.

Consider relaxation as yet another exercise that is an essential component of your fitness program. You need the active component, and you need the passive component. Without both, your fitness program is not whole, and you will not achieve the maximum benefits you seek—to get done as much as necessary and to get done the things you want to do.

9 Putting Your Exercise Program Together

Once you have reached the important decision to get fit, you next have to set about doing it. That means that you have to plan what you are going to do. You will need an exercise program that you can follow. If you belong to a facility that has an exercise professional, he or she should be able to help you plan such a program. Don't think that the exercise leader will set up a superjock program for you. Far from it. A professional should be able to tailor a program just for your needs in concert with the condition of your body. Still, you can plan your own program simply by applying the basic principles set forth in this chapter.

First of all, you have to know your function goals. You have to decide what you need to be fit for—what you want to do or do better and more easily.

You will also need to be aware of all aspects of your physical condition—your body's capacities and limitations, including the state of your physical fitness and health and any diseases or medical syndromes you may have. Your doctor can help delineate these for you based on your medical history and the tests given to you in preparation for starting your fitness program. Knowing these factors, you can decide which exercises to include in your program.

You have to take into account the access and availability of physical facilities, such as gyms and swimming pools, that may be useful in your program.

You also have to include two time factors. One of these is the scheduling time. Which times of the day, and which days, for exercising fit in best with your lifestyle? What hours and days are the facilities available to you? The other time factor is the long-range one. You need to be determined that exercising is a permanent part of your weekly routine.

Finally, you need patience. You need to realize that the benefits of exercise to your health and to your functioning will come slowly in

Physical activity plays an important role in preventing loss of human functional capacity with age. Each system of the human body has demonstrated an enhanced functional capacity through physical activity. The combination of increased physical activity and lifestyle modification will enable the older adult to enjoy a high quality of life.
—Everett L. Smith, Ph.D., University of Wisconsin

increments. You won't suddenly feel terrific and be able to do everything just because you started exercising. It doesn't work that way. But it does work. You have to give it time.

Having set your goals, and with all factors at hand, you are ready to sit down and design your exercise program.

Applying Exercise Principles

For maximum effectiveness, your program has to be based on the principles that support the six goals of exercise discussed in previous chapters.

Let's review them.

Cardiovascular Fitness

To achieve cardiovascular fitness, you have to (1) exercise or participate in a sport until you sweat and (2) keep up the sweat-producing activity for a while. But *do not* undertake such physical activities until and unless your physician tells you it is OK. And then the doctor should give you an exercise prescription so that you know exactly how intense an activity you can undertake.

Exercises for the heart should be

—brisk enough to raise the heartbeat

—sustained for fifteen to thirty minutes at a session

—regular, so as to be repeated at least three times a week

Perhaps the best activities for the heart are walking, swimming, and cycling.

Poor exercises for the heart include baseball, softball, football, volleyball, golf, and bowling. These are either low-level activities or moderate-level activities that are done sporadically.

Moderate heart exercises include bicycling, downhill (Alpine) skiing, basketball, calisthenics, field hockey, handball, racquetball, squash, soccer, singles tennis, swimming, and brisk walking. These activities are done continuously or nearly so.

Vigorous heart exercises include cross-country (Nordic) skiing, uphill hiking, ice hockey, jogging, running in place, stationary cycling, and jumping rope. These activities are at a high level of intensity that is fairly well sustained.

Flexibility

Flexibility is the ability to move your joints freely. You shouldn't expect to regain the flexibility you had when you were twenty, but you should be able to recover a decent amount of it.

Ironically, movement itself is the best treatment for stiffness. At first, any movements should be gentle and slow, especially if there is arthritis in the joint. As flexibility returns to your joints, you can try increasing the amount of each movement and the speed you move increment by increment.

You usually begin your workout routine with flexibility exercises, as they serve well the purpose of warming up. For maximum effect, flexibility exercises should be performed daily. You will never become as flexible and supple as a dancer, but you can use the dancer's example. Dancers get that way, and stay that way, only by doing flexibility exercises—not just once a day but several times a day.

Among the best exercises for flexibility are walking, cycling, swimming, dancing, yoga, and calisthenics.

Muscle Strength

Strength is the muscle's ability to exert force. Muscles develop strength by being challenged and loaded. Exercises for strength should be done every other day rather than every day. The best strengthening exercises pit muscle against an outside force such as a dumbbell or an exercise machine.

In building up the strength of your muscles, decide which specific muscles you want to load. Then increase the load over time. For example, this month add one pound and next month add two pounds. Whether the new load is an additional one pound or ten pounds, your muscles will respond, and you can again build up the amount of weight or force you are working them against.

Endurance

Endurance is the combined ability of body and muscles to keep those muscles doing whatever they are doing. It is a combination of development of the muscles and development of the cardiovascular and respiratory systems, which supply fuel to the muscles.

Endurance exercises require muscles to work against force in many repetitions over time. Among the best are walking, cycling, jogging, swimming, tennis, and calisthenics.

Endurance does not happen immediately. It takes time. You need to build it up patiently, a step at a time.

Because there is so much overlap between endurance exercises and those used to help the cardiovascular system, the same caution applies: *Do not* undertake any vigorous physical activities until you have seen your physician and obtained an exercise prescription.

Leanness

Exercise helps in slimming in three ways:

1. It curbs appetite, so you don't eat as many calories as before.

2. It burns off calories, so you lose fat.

3. It firms up the flesh left behind after your weight loss.

The only part of your body you can spot-reduce is your tummy. Exercise won't take away the fat under the abdominal wall, but it can reduce the layer of fat between the abdominal wall and your skin. The best exercises for tightening your tummy are sit-ups, head curls, leg raises, walking, and jogging.

Slimming requires you to repeat each exercise many times and do the same exercises every day.

Relaxation

The best methods for relaxation are any exercises that wear you out, progressive relaxation, meditation, yoga, and massage.

You will find that your muscles want very much to relax after they have been worked out. Listen to them. Always schedule times for relaxation in your workout program. This can be as simple as sitting in a sauna or being massaged. Or it can be relaxing progressively, meditating, or doing some yoga.

In progressive relaxation, you start at the feet and work up to your head, tensing and then ultrarelaxing each set of muscles. In meditation, you merely concentrate on one thing. In yoga, you perform certain body movements gently.

Getting Your Act Together

It's time to put all the pieces into a program, or get your act together. Start by reviewing the Functional Fitness Self-Assessment you should have completed in chapter 3. If you did not take it when you read that chapter, this is a good time to complete it.

Having taken the Functional Fitness Self-Assessment, you should have a rather clear picture of your flexibility, strength, endurance, and body fat. And you should have not only the Big Picture but also details of the picture. In other words, you should know which areas of your body have more and which less of each aspect of physical fitness. In order to improve those areas with less, you need to program the appropriate exercises. And you need to design your program so that you can reasonably and effectively improve upon the condition you are now in, stage by stage, until you reach the level that serves your purpose.

To put your program together properly, you will need to know more about specific exercises at specific levels of intensity for specific functions. These details appear in chapters 10 through 13. Knowing what level you are at, you can select the exercises you need from the appropriate chapter. They are organized in this way.

Exercises at the Low-Intensity Level

These are exercises for the person at the Minimum Fitness Level who is just starting to exercise for the first time in his or her life or after many, many years. They are also for the person whose motions are limited by arthritis.

Exercises at the Low-Medium Intensity Level

These are exercises for the person at the Poor Fitness Level. This is most likely someone who has been sedentary for years, mildly active once in a while, and now wants to become active.

Exercises at the Medium-Intensity Level

These are exercises for the person at the Average Fitness Level. This is most likely someone who has been mildly active but who wants to be more active, even mildly athletic.

Exercises at the High-Intensity Level

These are exercises for the person at the Very Good Fitness Level. This is most likely someone who is already in good physical shape and who wants to get into active, even competitive, sports.

Two Examples

So far, the discussion of program design has been rather abstract. Let's get practical with two examples.

Case: The Nine-to-Fiver

GOALS: To lose weight. To decrease the risk of heart attack.
FITNESS LEVEL: Average
LIMITATIONS: Overweight
EXERCISES: (from chapter 12)
    for leanness, every day:
        Head Curl, twenty-five times
        Side Leg Raise, twenty times each side
        Standing Crawl, five minutes
    for cardiovascular health, three times a week:
        Swimming Crawl, twenty minutes
        Walking, start at one mile, build up to two miles, and then
            add ten jog steps for every fifty walk steps.

COMMENTS: Exercise is a great way to wake up before your morning shower. You'll feel stimulated when you get to work. If you have a pool handy, do the crawl in the water after work. It helps get the muscle kinks out. If you are serious about losing weight, you'll also have to cut back on your daily consumption of calories.

Case: The Retiree

Suppose that (like many of us) you have been sedentary for as long as you can remember, and now you have decided that it is time to get active and get into shape. Suppose, too, that (like many of us) you have a little arthritis in your shoulders.

Here's what your program would look like.

GOAL: To be able to bicycle to the supermarket a mile away whenever I wish.

FITNESS LEVEL: Poor

LIMITATIONS: Arthritis in shoulder.

Not in shape.

Nearest YMCA five miles away with exercise rooms open in the afternoon.

EXERCISES: (from chapter 11)

for flexibility, every day:

Main Street Stroll and Twist, three minutes

Arm Circle, five times in each circular direction

Flexed-Leg Forward Bend, five times

Raised-Knee Crossover, five times

for muscle strength, three times a week:

Half Knee Bend, six times

Knee-up, five times

for endurance, every other day:

Walking, twenty minutes at faster than normal pace.

COMMENTS: You will have to exercise in the afternoon. Just make sure that you wait at least an hour after lunch. If you feel fatigued or faint at any time during your workout, slow down. Also, you'll have to drive to the Y, get a ride, or take a bus. Later, when your endurance and strength are up, and the weather is good, you should be able to bicycle there.

The above example is addressed to but one goal. However, in putting together your own personal program, you may have as many goals as you wish. To continue the example above, you may decide that in addition to being able to cycle to the supermarket, you also want to start playing tennis, to be able to swim a quarter of a mile, to start learning cabinetmaking, and to attend weekly social dances. You *can* do all that if you get yourself into fitness. This requires that you regularly follow a program that includes all the exercises necessary to support the activities that you like so much.

The Exercises

Here is a list of all the exercises in this book, indicating the purpose of the exercise, the level of intensity, and the muscular area benefited. This information and the descriptions of the exercises in chapters 10 to 13 will help you design your exercise program in relation to what the exercises do and what your fitness goals are, and then carry it out.

Cardiovascular Fitness

Low-Medium Intensity

Exercise:	*Muscles:*
Jogging in Place	heart, lung
Walking	heart, lung

Medium Intensity

Exercise:	*Muscles:*
Swimming Crawl	heart, lung
Walking-Jogging	heart, lung

High Intensity

Exercise:	*Muscles:*
Stair Climbing	heart, lung
Rope Skipping	heart, lung
Dancing	heart, lung
Walking-Jogging	heart, lung
Cycling	heart, lung
Nordic (X-C) Skiing	heart, lung
Rowing	heart, lung
High Bobbing	heart, lung
Advanced Treading	heart, lung
Lap Swimming	heart, lung

Flexibility

Low Intensity

Exercise:	*Muscles:*
Head Roll	neck, shoulder
Head Bob	neck
Arm Circle	shoulder, elbow
Hand Exercise	hand, wrist
Seated Triangle	trunk
Front Slump	back
Side Bend	trunk
Ankle Exercise	ankle, lower leg
Knee Lift	abdomen, hip, knee
Sitting Stretch	back
Toe Bounce	leg, ankle
Flutter Kick	back, hip, leg

Low-Medium Intensity

Exercise:	*Muscles:*
Main Street Stroll and Twist	shoulder, trunk, arm, leg
Head Roll	neck, shoulder
Arm Circle	shoulder, elbow
Wing Stretcher	shoulder, upper back, chest, arm

Body Side-Bender	trunk, arm, leg
Flexed-Leg Forward Bend	back, hip, leg
Flutter Kick	back, hip, leg
Standing Crawl	shoulder, back, arm
Knee-up	hip, knee
Raised-Knee Crossover	trunk, hip, knee

Medium Intensity

Exercise:	*Muscles:*
Main Street Stroll and Twist	shoulder, trunk, arm, leg
Head Roll	neck, shoulder
Arm Circle	shoulder, elbow
Wing Stretcher	shoulder, upper back, chest, arm
Body Side-Bender	trunk, arm, leg
Flexed-Leg Forward Bend	back, hip, leg
Flutter Kick	back, hip, leg
Raised-Knee Crossover	trunk, hip, knee
Swimming Crawl	neck, shoulder, arm, trunk, leg

High Intensity

Exercise:	*Muscles:*
Main Street Stroll and Twist	shoulder, trunk, arm, leg
Arm Propeller	shoulder, elbow, wrist
Wing Stretcher	shoulder, upper back, chest, arm
Body Side-Bender	trunk, arm, leg
Alternate Floor Touch	arm, trunk, back of leg
Sitting Stretch	arm, back, back of leg
Side Leg Raise and Whip	hip, thigh
Leg Stretch	back of thigh, back of ankle
Knee Raise and Hug	hip, knee
Flutter Kick	back, hip, leg
Sprinter	back, back of leg
Raised-Knee Crossover	trunk, hip, knee
Lap Swimming	neck, shoulder, arm, trunk, leg

Muscle Strength

Low Intensity

Exercise:	*Muscles:*
Arm Circle	shoulder, arm
Hand Exercise	lower arm
Tummy Tightener	abdomen
Leg Extension	front of thigh, groin

Thigh Toner	inner thigh, outer thigh
Thigh Strengthener	front of thigh
Rear Leg Raise	buttock, hip, back of leg
Side Leg Raise	hip, trunk
Head Curl	upper abdomen
Flutter Kick	lower abdomen

Low-Medium Intensity

Exercise:	*Muscles:*
Arm Circle	shoulder, arm
Wing Stretcher	upper back, shoulder, arm
Chest Press-Pull	shoulder, chest, arm
Half Knee Bend	front of thigh
Heel Raise	calf, ankle, arch
Head Curl	upper abdomen
Leg Lift	lower abdomen, front of thigh
Side Leg Raise	hip, outer thigh
Knee Push-up	arm, shoulder, chest, abdomen
Flutter Kick	neck, back, buttock, back of thigh
Knee-up	lower abdomen, hip, front of thigh
Raised-Knee Crossover	lower abdomen
Jogging in Place	hip, leg, foot

Medium Intensity

Exercise:	*Muscles:*
Head Roll	neck, shoulder, arm
Arm Circle	shoulder, arm
Wing Stretcher	upper back, shoulder, arm
Chest Press-Pull	shoulder, chest, arm
Half Knee Bend	front of thigh
Heel Raise	calf, ankle, arch
Head Curl	upper abdomen
Leg Lift	lower abdomen, front of thigh
Side Leg Raise	hip, outer thigh
Knee Push-up	arm, shoulder, chest, abdomen
Flutter Kick	neck, back, buttock, back of thigh
Raised-Knee Crossover	lower abdomen
Treading Water	lower abdomen, leg
Swimming Crawl	all

High Intensity

Exercise:	*Muscles:*
Wing Stretcher	shoulder, upper back
Chest Press-Pull	shoulder, chest, arm
Samson Door Press	shoulder, upper back, upper arm
Squat	thigh
Heel Raise	calf, ankle, arch
Arm Curl	upper arm, hand
Arm Extension	shoulder, upper arm, hand
Chest Fly	shoulder, chest
Head Curl	upper abdomen
Side Leg Raise and Whip	waist ("love handles")
Knee Raise and Hug	hip, knee
Flutter Kick	neck, back, buttock, back of thigh
Sit-up	abdomen
Push-up	shoulder, chest, abdomen
Raised-Knee Crossover	lower abdomen, thigh
Nordic (X-C) Skiing	arm, leg
Advanced Treading	lower abdomen, leg
Lap Swimming	all

Endurance

Low Intensity

Exercise:	*Muscles:*
Walking	hip, leg, foot

Low-Medium Intensity

Exercise:	*Muscles:*
Side-Straddle Hop	arm, leg
Jogging in Place	leg
Walking	hip, leg, foot

Medium Intensity

Exercise:	*Muscles:*
Side-Straddle Hop	arm, leg
Walking-Jogging	hip, leg, foot
Bob	leg
Treading Water	lower abdomen, leg
Swimming Crawl	all

High Intensity

Exercise:	*Muscles:*
Side-Straddle Hop	arm, leg
Rowing	shoulder, arm
Stair Climbing	thigh

Rope Skipping	leg, foot
Walking-Jogging	hip, leg, foot
Dancing	leg, foot
Cycling	leg
Nordic (X-C) Skiing	arm, leg
High Bobbing	arm, leg
Advanced Treading	lower abdomen, leg
Lap Swimming	all

Leanness

Low Intensity

Exercise:	*Muscles:*
Tummy Tightener	abdomen
Head Curl	upper abdomen

Low-Medium Intensity

Exercise:	*Muscles:*
Head Curl	upper abdomen
Side Leg Raise	waist ("love handles")

Medium Intensity

Exercise:	*Muscles:*
Head Curl	upper abdomen
Side Leg Raise	waist ("love handles")
Swimming Crawl	all

High Intensity

Exercise:	*Muscles:*
Head Curl	upper abdomen
Side Leg Raise and Whip	waist ("love handles")
Lap Swimming	all

Relaxation

Exercise:	*Muscles:*
Humming Breath	mouth, throat
Seated Sun Salutation	back
Front Slump	back
Seated Triangle	trunk
Head Roll	neck, shoulder
Head Bob	neck
Hand Exercise	hand, wrist
Arm Circle	shoulder, elbow
Phoenix	neck, back, arm, buttock
Lap Swimming	all

The guide that follows will help you design your Fitness for Life exercise program.

It is structured to help you think through your fitness goals and translate them into an exercise program that can help you achieve those goals. It is meant to be used with the exercise list on pages 62–67, which is organized by purpose, levels of intensity, and areas of the body benefited.

**My
Fitness for Life
Exercise Program**

My fitness level: _____

My fitness goals:

1. _____
2. _____
3. _____
4. _____
5. _____

My limitations:

1. _____
2. _____
3. _____
4. _____
5. _____

Exercises and repetitions that can help me accomplish my goals:

1. _____
2. _____
3. _____
4. _____
5. _____
6. _____
7. _____
8. _____
9. _____
10. _____
11. _____

12. _____
13. _____
14. _____
15. _____
16. _____
17. _____
18. _____
19. _____
20. _____
21. _____
22. _____
23. _____
24. _____
25. _____
26. _____
27. _____
28. _____
29. _____
30. _____

Sports, and duration of play, that can help me accomplish my cardiovascular and endurance fitness goals.

1. _____
2. _____
3. _____
4. _____
5. _____

Following is a chart for keeping track of your exercise efforts and accomplishments.

My Workout Week

Goals: _____ minutes of exercise per day
          _____ average daily reduction in calories

MONDAY: Time   Place   Exercises _____
_____

Comments (note any changes in intensity level and any goals achieved):
_____
_____

TUESDAY: Time   Place   Exercises _____
_____

Comments: _____

WEDNESDAY: Time   Place   Exercises _____
_____

Comments: _____

THURSDAY: Time   Place   Exercises _____
_____

Comments: _____

FRIDAY: Time   Place   Exercises _____
_____

Comments: _____

SATURDAY: Time   Place   Exercises _____
_____

Comments: _____

SUNDAY: Time   Place   Exercises _____
_____

Comments: _____

10 Exercises at the Low-Intensity Level

These low-intensity exercises are characterized by gentle, slow movements. Their main purpose is to increase the flexibility of limbs, trunk, and neck and to begin strengthening the major muscles of the body.

Another purpose of these exercises is to help you relax.

A final purpose is to help you get started on the road to fitness. As the old Chinese adage says, Even a journey of a thousand miles begins with the first step.

You belong at this level if any of the following statements is true.

- You scored very low (0 to 14 points) on the fitness assessment in chapter 3.

- You have never had an exercise program (having held a job for years or had a hobby that kept you on your feet or otherwise active doesn't count, as it was certainly not a well-rounded exercise program that covered all possible and desirable goals).

- You have not been in good physical shape for years.

- You have severe arthritis or another physical condition that limits your flexibility and ability to move.

- You want to, or have to, exercise in a chair or in bed. (Be aware that six of the exercises, beginning with exercise 13, require standing.)

While some of these twenty exercises are derived from yoga, they are *not* meant to be performed to the limit of any joint's range of motion or to get you into any awkward postures or contortions. They are not intended to cause you pain. They should exercise but not tax your muscles, tendons, ligaments, joints, heart, lungs, or any other part of your body. For these reasons, they are not well suited to achieving the goals of cardiovascular fitness, muscle strength, endurance, and leanness. But, then, you are not ready for those goals yet.

Wherever there is muscle there is need of movement. . . . Proper exercise . . . prolongs your active years.
—President's Council on Physical Fitness and Sports

71

Remember, if you have not exercised in years, or ever, you must check with your doctor before including these exercises in your personal fitness program. That goes double if you have not been in good physical health for years.

So that you will know how this program will start you toward your fitness goals, each of the twenty exercises described here is coded. As you can see, the code refers to goals.

F = Flexibility
S = Strength
E = Endurance

You will note that the twenty exercises are presented in the order in which they are to be done, from the head down.

Your body warms up more efficiently when you exercise in the order of small to large muscles. The muscles of your legs are the largest in your body.

Exercises 1 through 11 can be done in the sitting position. If you have easy access to a swimming pool, you should consider doing exercises 9, 11, 12, 13, 14, 18, and 19 at the shallow end, holding on to the edge as necessary.

Each of the exercises in this program initially calls for five repetitions. After you have been on this program for a week or two, increase the number to ten. After another week or two, increase to fifteen. Then keep it there.

You should repeat this program of exercises at least three times a week in order for your body to get maximum benefit. Every day would be even better. If you have no easy access to a pool, do all the exercises in a chair and on the floor.

The exercises are on the pages that follow.

1. Head Roll. Slowly roll your head around in a circle, through its entire range of motion. Start by dropping it toward your chest. Then rotate it toward your shoulder, then toward your back, then toward the opposite shoulder, and finally forward again. Go in a clockwise direction five times and then in a counterclockwise direction five times to relax your neck muscles. As your head revolves, close your eyes and try to simultaneously relax those neck muscles, as well as the muscles in your shoulders. (F)

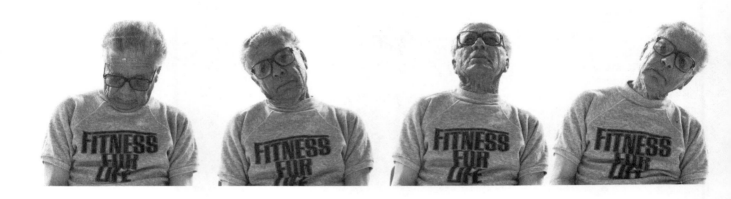

2. Head Bob. Let your head drop forward *slowly,* and push it gently down a little more as you try to touch your chin to your chest. Hold it for a count of three. Then slowly raise your head back to its usual erect position, and let it fall backward (slowly). Again, push it a bit, but gently. Hold it for a count of three; then bring it back to its usual erect position. Do this five times to limber up your neck. (F)

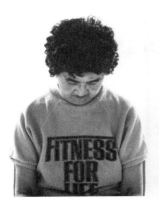
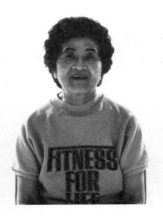
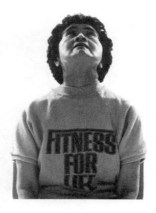

Moving Up

Mastering these low-intensity exercises may take a month to three months, depending on your body and on your diligence. Then you may want to consider moving up to the next intensity level, low-medium. And, when you have mastered that level, you may want to move up again, to medium, and so on. That's up to you.

The results of the Functional Fitness Self-Assessment (see chapter 3), your own sense of what you physically can and cannot do, and your desire to do more will determine which fitness level is best for you. You alone are the master or mistress of your fate. You alone must know what you want to go for and what you can go for. You alone must plan the goals of your fitness program in terms of the functions you want to achieve. Those goals will tell you which exercise level to strive for.

3. Arm Circle.   Raise your arms to a T position—extended to the sides, at shoulder height. Make fists with your hands. Tighten the elbows and muscles of your arms and make small circular motions, keeping your arms rigid. Make five rotations in one direction, five in the opposite direction. *Then* relax your hands and elbow, and make large circles with your arms still extended. Rotate five times in one direction and five times in the opposite direction to loosen your shoulders and elbows. (F, S)

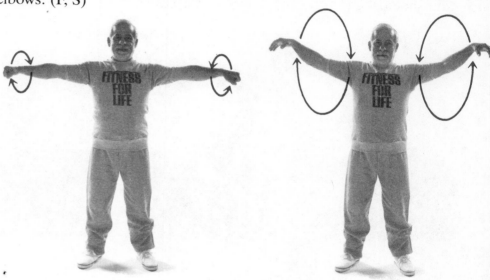

4. Hand Exercises.   With your arms extended as in exercise 3, above, tighten and then relax your fists. Do this five times. Let the hands flop down, relaxed; then raise them. Do this five times. Finally, describe circles with your hands at the wrists, five times in each direction, to loosen your wrists. (F, S)

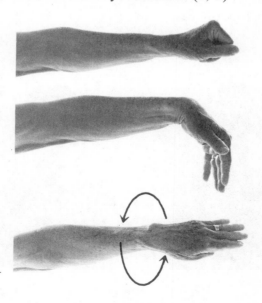

5. Seated Triangle.   As you sit in a chair, your hips facing forward, raise your arms to a T position. Inhale deeply. Now exhale, and as you do so, slowly move the right hand down to the toes of your left foot. Remember to keep the T so that as you rotate your trunk, your left arm follows the movement and rotates until it is pointing to the ceiling. Turn your head to the left so that you can look at the left thumb. Hold that position for five seconds. Inhale and come back to the original upright T position. Alternate five left and five right toe touches to loosen your trunk. (F)

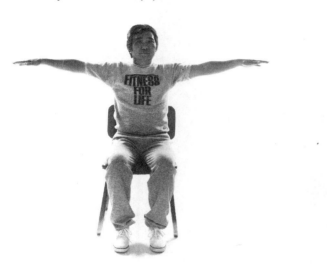 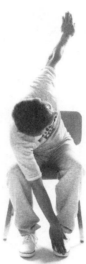

6. Front Slump.   Sitting so that your buttocks are firmly against the back of a hard chair, slump your shoulders and head, and let your arms drop to the sides. Now let your upper body slump down, bending slowly at the waist so that your chest is in your lap and your fingers are touching the floor. Hold for a few seconds; then s-l-o-w-l-y raise yourself to the upright sitting position. Tighten your abdominal muscles as you do so. Do this five times to limber the long muscles that run down your spine. (F)

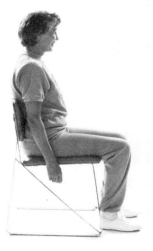 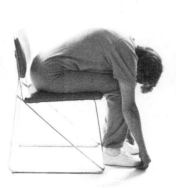 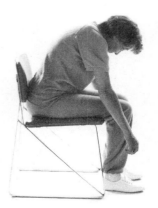

7. Tummy Tightener.   This can be done from the sitting position at any time. Do it whenever you think about it—when you are on the phone, when you are driving and are stopped at a traffic light, when you are sitting down to a cup of coffee. Sitting in a chair, contract your abdominal muscles as hard as you can. Try to hold this for about half a minute. Relax; let your tummy come forward by itself; then push it forward and hold. Do this five times. Strenghtening those sagging abdominal muscles will not only firm them but will help your back as well. (S)

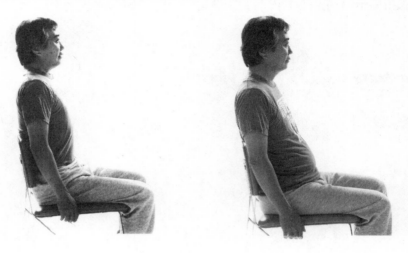

8. Side Bend.   Still sitting, let your hands hang down your sides. Drop your body from the waist up, to the left. Try to touch the fingertips of the left hand to the floor. Bring yourself back up to a full sitting position; then drop to the right side. Bring yourself back up. Alternate sides five times to loosen your trunk muscles. (F)

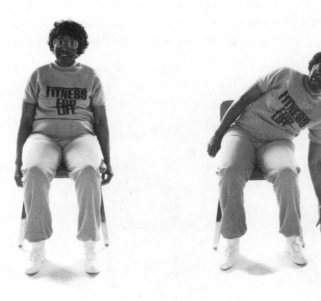

9. Leg Extension. Sitting, lift your left leg off the floor, and extend it fully in front of you. Hold it for the count of five; then slowly lower it. Do the same with the right leg. Do five of each leg to tone the thigh muscles. (S)

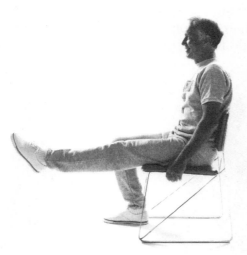

10. Thigh Toner. Sitting, lean forward and place each hand at the outside of its respective (left or right) knee. As you slowly try to separate the thighs, use your hands to keep the thighs together. Count to five and relax. Do this five times. Next, place your hands on the insides of your knees, and use your hands to oppose the thighs as you try to close them. Again, count to five at each attempt, and repeat five times to tone the inner and outer thigh muscles. (S)

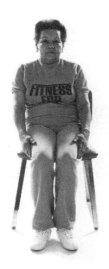 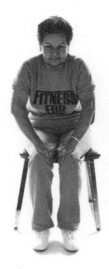

11. Ankle Exercise.   Sitting, lift both legs off the floor, slightly apart. Move your feet to four positions, in this order: (1) point the toes inward, toward each other; (2) point them outward, away from each other; (3) point them up, toward you; and (4) point them down, away from you. Hold in each of the four positions for the count of five. Do five sets, as hard as you can. It may help to hold on to the seat of the chair as you do this exercise. (F)

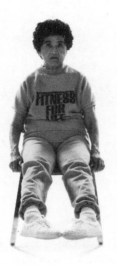
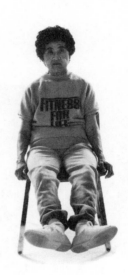

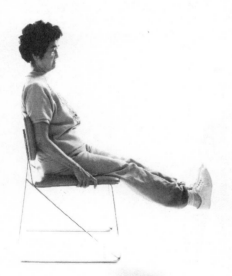
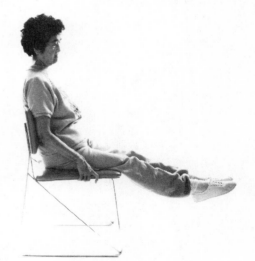

12. Thigh Strengthener. Arms hanging loosely at your sides, slowly lift yourself from a sitting position to a standing position. After a count of five, slowly lower yourself back to a sitting position, keeping your back as straight as you can. As you do so, hold your loose-hanging hands slightly behind you so that you can feel the seat of the chair behind you to assure that you do not miss it as you sit. (S)

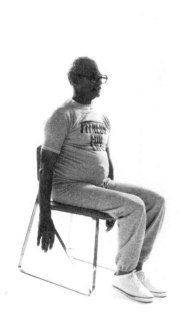
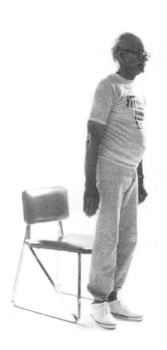
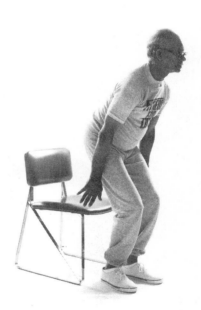

13. Rear Leg Raise.   Feet together, stand behind your chair, facing it. Grasp the back. Lift your left leg back, and raise it as high as you can. Try to keep your knee straight. Slowly lower your leg back down to the floor. Do the same with your right leg. Repeat five times to help firm your buttocks, strengthen the lower back, and limber your hips and legs. (F, S)

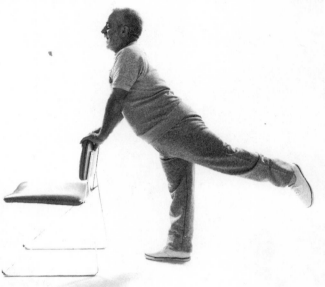

14. Knee Lift.   Feet together, stand behind your chair, the chair at your right side. Grasp the back of the chair with your right hand, and raise your left knee as high as you can in front of you. Repeat five times; then turn around and hold on to the chair with your left hand. Raise the right knee five times to help tone up your knees, hips, and lower abdomen. (F)

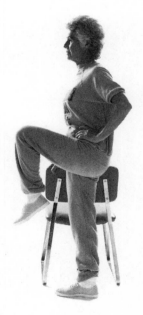

15. Sitting Stretch.   Sit on a carpet or mat, with your hands balancing you at your sides and slightly behind you. Spread your legs. Slowly stretch forward at the waist, and extend your arms forward as far as you can. Hold for three seconds or so. Return to a full sitting position. Repeat five times. (F)

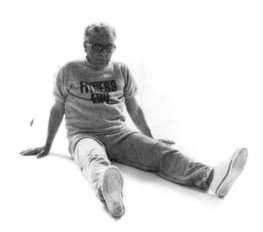 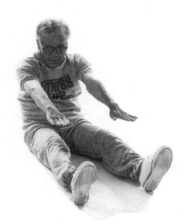

16. Side Leg Raise.   Lie on your left side, with your head resting on your left arm, which is extended past your head, and your right hand on the floor in front of your abdomen to balance you. Lift your right leg sideward as high as you can. Hold it for a count of two. Repeat five times; then roll over and raise the left leg five times to help tone your hip muscles and trunk muscles. (S)

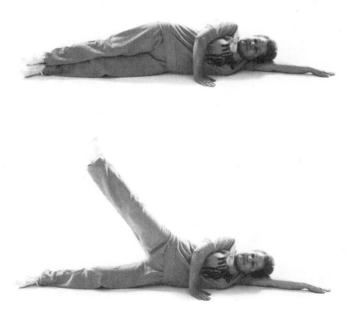

17. Head Curl. Lie on your back, with your legs stretched out and together. Stretch your arms along the front of your body, with your palms resting on the front of your thighs. Raise your head and shoulders as far forward as you can. As you do so, let your hands slide down your thighs with your arms still extended. Hold for a count of three; then slowly let your head back down to the carpet or mat. Relax for a count of three. Repeat five times to tighten your neck and abdominal muscles. (S)

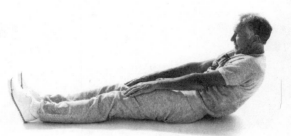

Pain and Injury

When you exercise, "listen" to your body. Pain is one way it communicates. Pain is a non-verbal message. When the message is fairly quiet and somewhat nagging, it likely means that some structure has been stressed. You should then slow down or ease back.

An example of such pain is the muscle soreness you may feel the day after each exercise session during the first weeks of your exercise program. Warm baths, massage, and liniment help ease the soreness. Reduced pace and twenty-four hours of rest help more.

A message loud and very painful may mean you have a serious condition. In any case, your first action should be to stop—now!

The simplest treatment is to elevate the affected area above the level of the heart. This elevation acts to prevent or minimize swelling.

Next, apply cold, preferably from ice wrapped in cloth or plastic.

Any pain that lasts more than a few days needs to be discussed with your physician. It might be telling you of a serious injury.

18. Toe Bounce. Standing, holding on to the back of a chair, slowly raise yourself on your toes. If you have access to a pool, stand in chest-high water, place your hands on your hips, and jump up with both feet in a slow, bouncing movement. On land or in the pool, try to keep your knees straight and use only your toes. Do five times, and then rest. Do two more sets of five to limber and warm up. (S)

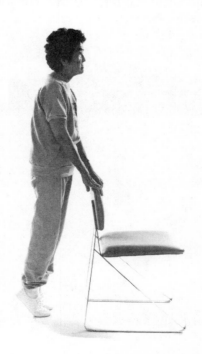

19. Flutter Kick. On your back on a mat or carpet, kick your legs in a flutter. Make sure your legs are up and your knees are bent so as to protect your back. If you have access to a pool, hold on to the sides of the pool with both hands behind you so that your back is in the water, your front is facing up, and your head is out of the water, facing your toes. (Do not do on land if you have a bad back.) On land or in the water, do this five times to limber your legs and feet and strengthen your abdominal muscles. (F, S)

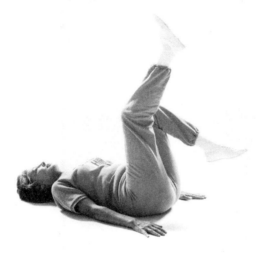

20. Walking. Next to swimming, the best exercise at every level of intensity is walking. At this level start out by walking a third of a mile. If it takes you about six minutes, fine; that's about three miles per hour. If it takes you twelve minutes, that's OK, too; that's about two miles per hour. Try to walk on smooth, level ground. Dress comfortably, and make sure you wear a good pair of walking or jogging shoes. If you feel uncomfortable, nauseated, or out of breath at any point along the way, stop and sit down for a while, until you feel better. After you feel you have mastered a third of a mile, try half a mile, then a whole mile. Over the next few weeks, too, try to increase the pace of your walking, which exercises your hips, your legs, and your feet. The massaging action of the muscles helps the veins of the legs move blood back to your heart, which is also exercised by walking. (S, E)

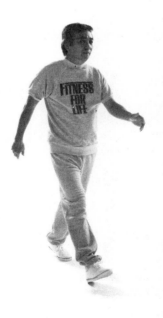

Always finish an exercise session by cooling down. One of the best cool-downs is a short, casual walk for five minutes. No stress, no hurry. Do not go immediately to the shower, as you will then keep on sweating even after you towel down. Rather, wrap yourself in a towel or robe until you have stopped sweating; *then* go to the shower and enjoy the relaxation you've earned.

———————————

After a month or so at this low-intensity level, you might be ready to progress to the next intensity level, low-medium.

11 Exercises at the Low-Medium Intensity Level

Consider these twenty exercises if for the last few years you have led a sedentary life or otherwise have been out of shape and want to get back into shape, have a low score on the Functional Fitness Self-Assessment, or have mild arthritis.

If you are in good health and are interested in getting on the road to the peak of good physical shape, consider this your first leg of the trip. The road will climb and take increasing effort on your part but will bring you to new heights of fitness. At the new heights will be new abilities to do the things you want to do in your life—in other words, functional fitness.

Now that you have reached the first plateau, you will feel better about yourself and your new fitness than you have in a long time and likely better than you ever have before.

No one else can do it for you; no one else can put out the effort that is required but you. Still, you do not have to travel the fitness road alone. You may find that it is more pleasant to exercise with friends who are similarly interested in physical fitness than to exercise alone.

These exercises at low-medium intensity are characterized by somewhat gentle-to-moderate, slow-to-medium speed movements, with some mild stress and endurance components. Their main purpose is to provide some modest cardiovascular benefit, increase the flexibility of your joints, strengthen the major muscles of your body, increase your endurance, and start firming you up.

You should not experience pain in this program, though you will feel some stretching and other signs that you are doing physical work. You may also experience some mild muscle soreness the day after exercising, which is a good indication that you are pushing your body to new efforts.

The way to keep lively is to be lively; the way to stay active is to move. Energy begets energy, and the only way to develop the capacity to expend more and more energy is to keep increasingly active.
—Administration on Aging

85

So that you will know how this program will start you toward your fitness goals, each of the twenty exercises described here is coded. As you can see, the code refers to goals.

CV = Cardiovascular Fitness
F = Flexibility
S = Strength
E = Endurance
L = Leanness/Slimming
R = Relaxation

It is a good idea to do the exercises in the order in which they are presented here. The muscles of the head and neck are first to be exercised, and those of the feet are the last, with the muscles of the arms and trunk in between. More importantly, the exercises begin with smaller muscles and proceed to larger muscles (leg muscles are the biggest in your body). This gives the body a chance to gear up and progress from work to harder work to still harder work. Safe exercising relies upon the body warming up to bigger and bigger tasks rather than being given big tasks right at the start.

You should repeat your program of exercises at least three times a week. Of course, your weekly cycle of exercising depends on your goals. For maximum results, muscle-strengthening exercises should be done every other day, while all the others should be done daily.

Your exercising schedule will depend in large part on the availability of facilities and equipment and in small part on the cooperation of the weather. Five of the exercises can be done in a pool; these exercises are also tailored for dry land. If a pool is not available or if access is not convenient, do the next best thing.

The exercises begin at low levels of intensity (such as five repetitions) and build up to medium intensity (such as twenty repetitions). Stay with this plan, and after a month or so you should be at medium levels of intensity on most exercises.

The exercises are on the pages that follow.

1. Main Street Stroll and Twist. Simply walk around for three minutes on a level surface. Indoors is OK, but outdoors is even better. Breathe deeply. During the first minute, walk with an exaggerated swing in your arms, forward and backward. The second minute, raise your arms as you walk, and put them through swimming-the-crawl motions. The third minute, clasp your hands behind your head, and walk with an exaggerated twist of the shoulders—left and then right, and so on. Keep your hips stable in this warm-up exercise that limbers most of your body. It is best to do this exercise daily. After a week, increase to six minutes. (F)

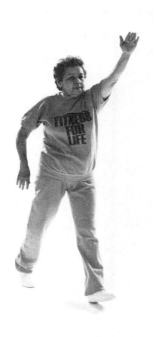
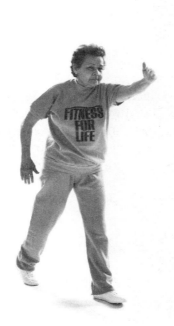
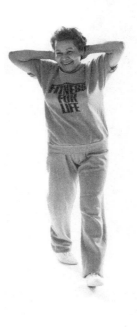

Breathe Deeply!
You must always breathe deeply when you exercise. Endurance activities will automatically force you to do this, but exercises at a lower intensity will not.

So you have to consciously breathe deeply.

As a guide, *exhale* strongly on exertion and *inhale* deeply at rest at every set of every exercise.

2. Head Roll.   Standing, with legs spread and hands on hips, slowly roll your head around in a circle through its entire range of motion. Begin by gently dropping your head forward, to your chest; then rotate it to the left shoulder, then to your back, then to the right shoulder, then forward. Close your eyes, and try to relax your shoulders as you revolve your head five times clockwise and five times counterclockwise to limber those tight neck muscles and joints. After doing this daily for a week, increase to ten revolutions in each direction. (F)

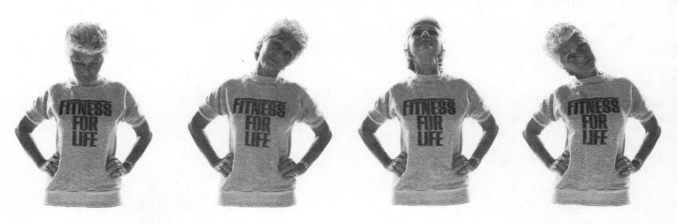

3. Arm Circle.   Standing, legs apart, raise both arms at shoulder height to a T position. Make fists with your hands, and tighten the elbows. Then make small circles, keeping your arms rigid. Revolve five times in forward circles, then five times in backward circles. After that, relax your hands and elbows and make large circles with your still-

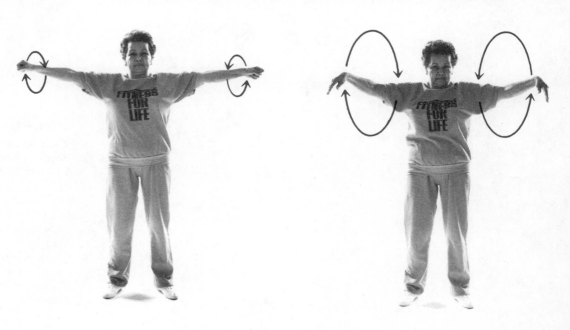

extended arms. Revolve five times in big forward circles and five times in big back circles to limber your shoulders and arms. After doing this daily for a week, increase to ten times each set. After two weeks, increase to fifteen times each set, and keep the repetitions at that level daily. (F, S)

4. Wing Stretcher. Standing, legs apart, arms straight out to the sides at T position, bend at the elbow to bring your hands to your chest, palms down, with your fingertips touching. This is a four-count exercise. On each count of 1-2-3, pull your elbows back as far as you can. Keep your arms at shoulder height as you pull back three times; then, on count 4, swing your hands all the way, straight out to the sides, turning your palms up. Return to the starting fingertip position. Do this five times every day for a week. In the second week, increase to ten to limber and strengthen your upper back, shoulders, arms, and chest and to improve your posture. (F, S)

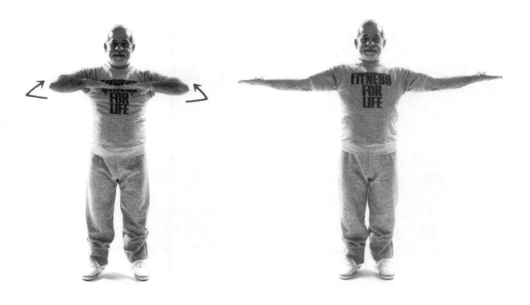

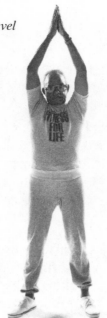
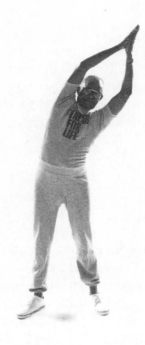

5. Body Side-Bender.   Standing, legs apart, feet spaced as wide as your shoulders, extend your arms straight up, palms facing, fingertips touching. A four-count exercise: (1) bend sideways at the waist to the left as far as you can; (2) return to upright; (3) bend to the right; (4) return to the starting position. Try to keep your elbows straight. Bend smoothly without any jerks, and only as far as you comfortably can. Do five repetitions every day the first week. The second week, increase to seven, and try to move a little farther in each bend than you did in the first week. The third week, increase to ten, and try to move a little farther yet. Keep working at this level to stretch your arm and leg muscles and limber your trunk. (F)

6. Flexed-Leg Forward Bend.   Standing, feet apart, hold your arms straight over your head, thumbs laced. Flex (slightly bend) your knees as you bend forward at the waist. Keep the knees bent (to protect your lower back) as you extend your fingertips toward your left toes. Stretch gently. Not touching your toes is all right. Hold it there for the count of five; then stand up. Bend forward again and try to touch your right toes. Repeat five times. Next week do seven repetitions. The third week do ten and keep the exercise at this level every day to limber your back, hips, and legs. (F)

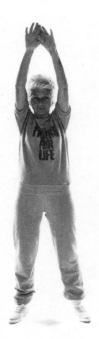
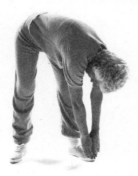

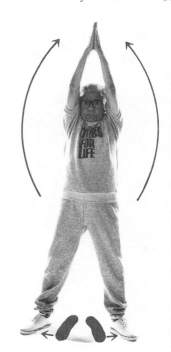

7. Side-Straddle Hop. Also known as a jumping jack, this exercise begins with you standing, feet together, hands hanging down at your sides. The actions of arms and legs in this two-count exercise are simultaneous: (1) Spread your legs in one jumping action as your hands come together over your head. Exhale as you do this. (2) Inhale as you jump back to the starting position. Do daily, five the first week, ten the second week, fifteen the third week, to tone your arms and legs and stimulate your breathing and heart to build endurance. (E)

8. Chest Press-Pull. Standing, feet apart, bring your arms to shoulder height, and bend them at the elbows so that your hands are in front of your chest. Inhale deeply. Exhale as you p-u-s-h your palms against each other. Keep pushing for the count of five. Then separate your hands, and hook the fingers of one hand with the fingers of the other. Inhale deeply. Exhale as you try to p-u-l-l your hooked fingers apart. Keep pulling for a count of five. Do five sets of pushes and pulls every other day for the first week, seven sets for the second week, ten for the third, to strengthen arm, shoulder, and chest muscles. (S)

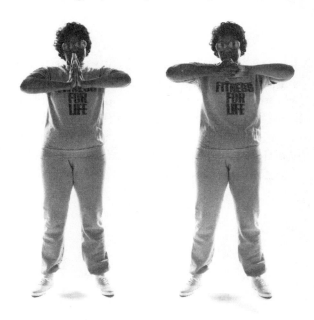

9. Half Knee Bend.   Standing, legs apart, place your hands on your hips. This is a two-count exercise: (1) lower your body halfway on bent knees as your arms extend forward, palms down; (2) rise, and return to the starting position. Move smoothly, keep your back straight, and breathe deeply. Exhale as you lower your body; inhale as you raise it. Do six bends every other day the first week, nine every other day the second week, and twelve every other day the third week, to strengthen your thigh muscles. (S)

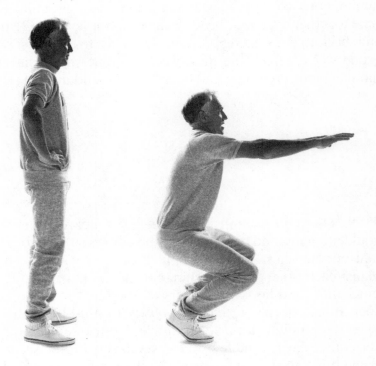

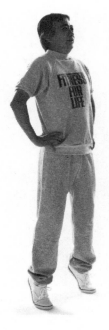

10. Heel Raise.   Standing, feet slightly apart, hands on hips, raise yourself so that you are standing on your toes; then lower yourself back to the floor. Do this as smoothly as you can. Inhale as you return to starting position; exhale as you raise up. Do four raises every other day the first week, eight each session the second week, twelve the third week, and sixteen the fourth week. Keep it at this level to strengthen your arches, ankles, and calves. (S)

11. Head Curl. Lying on your back on a carpet or mat, stretch out your legs, and hold them together. Tuck your hands, palms down, into the arch at the small of your back. Lift your head and shoulders, and elbows, off the floor. Hold for a count of five. You should feel a good tightness in your abdomen from the muscles holding up your head. Lower your head and shoulders, and elbows, back to the floor. Breathe deeply. Exhale on rising; inhale on relaxing. Do five every day the first week, ten every day the second week, and fifteen every day the third week. If you can build to twenty every day after that, all the better, since this is the best tummy-firming exercise. (L, S)

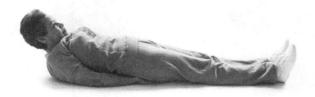

12. Leg Lift. Lying on your back on a carpet or mat, stretch out your legs, and hold them together. Place your hands under your hips, palms down. Raise your left leg, knee straight, off the floor. Hold it for a count of five. Then lower it back to the floor. Inhale deeply. Exhale as you raise the straightened right leg and hold for a count of five. Repeat five times every other day in the first week, ten every other day in the second week, and fifteen every other day in the third week, to strengthen the abdominal and front thigh muscles. (S)

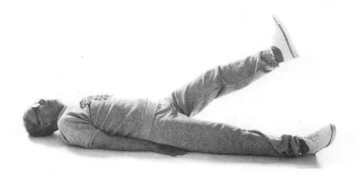

13. Side Leg Raise.   Lying on your left side on a carpet or mat, extend your straightened left arm in line with your body. Rest your head on the arm. Your right arm in front of you, palm on floor, helps balance you. Start with your legs together. Raise the straightened right leg as high as you can; then slowly lower it back to its original position. Do that ten times. Then roll over to your right side, and raise the left leg ten times. During the second week, raise each leg twenty times, and in the third week, thirty times. Done daily, this exercise strengthens hip and outer thigh muscles and slims down those "love handles" on your flanks. (S)

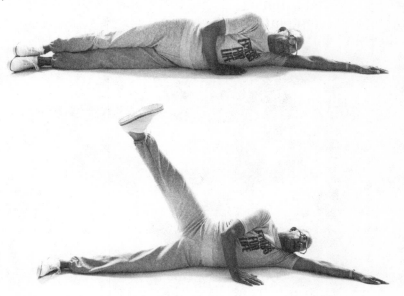

14. Knee Push-up.   Lying on your tummy, legs together, place your hands under your shoulders, palms on the floor. Bend your knees so that you raise your feet off the floor. Now, keeping your back straight, push against the floor until your arms are fully extended and your body, from the knees up, is off the floor. Slowly lower yourself to the floor, keeping your knees bent. Repeat five times. On the third week, increase to eight. On the fifth week, increase to twelve. Done every other day, this exercise strengthens arm, shoulder, chest, and abdominal muscles. (S)

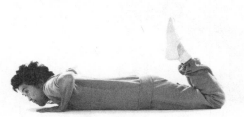
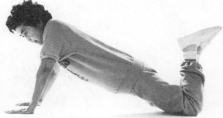

15. Flutter Kick.   This can be done on the floor or in a swimming pool. On the floor, lie facedown, and tuck your hands under your thighs. Arch your back so as to bring your head off the floor and your legs off the floor, toes pointed. Hold this position as you slightly separate your legs and kick them in a continuous flutter for thirty seconds. Over the next three weeks, work up to a full minute. The legs should kick from the hips, with the knees only slightly bent. In the swimming pool, lie with your front in the water, and hold on to the side of the pool. Point your toes, and kick in a whip action with knees and ankles flexible. On the floor or in the pool, breathe deeply. Do this thirty seconds daily now and a minute daily in three weeks to limber and strengthen your back, your buttocks, the back of your neck, and the backs of your thighs. (F, S)

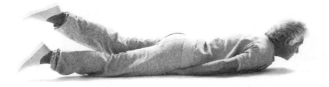

16. Standing Crawl.   Stand with your legs spread for stability. Bend forward and simulate the overhand crawl swimming stroke: Reach out with your left hand and dip into the "water." Get a "grip" on the "water," press downward, and pull your hand back to your shoulder; keep pulling the hand past your body. As your left hand comes by the left shoulder, your right hand should reach out. The same is true of the opposite hand. Keep the left and right hands working in a rhythm of opposition. Inhale on right-hand thrust; exhale on left. On days when a pool is handy, stand in chest-deep water and do it. On land and in the pool, make sure your legs are firmly planted, as balance is a problem when you are bending forward. This daily exercise is wonderful for limbering your arms, shoulders, and back and for improving coordination (F)

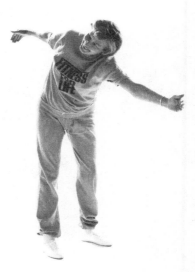

17. Knee-up.   Lying on your back, stretch your legs straight, feet together. Bring your knees up as tight to your chest as you can. With your knees up, gently swing your ankles to the left and then to the right; then stretch out. Exhale as you bring your knees up; inhale as you stretch out. Repeat five times every other day this week and ten times every other day next week to tone your abdomen, hips, and thighs. On days when the pool is handy, do this with your arms spread behind you, holding on to the edge. (F, S)

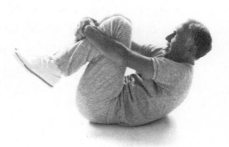

18. Raised-Knee Crossover.   Lie on your back, arms spread-eagle. Raise both knees together until your thighs are vertical; then swing them to the left as far as you can, trying to touch your knees to the floor. Then swing back to the center, and twist to the right as far as you can. Exhale deeply as you twist to the side; inhale as you return to the center position. On days when a pool is handy, stand in chest-deep water with your back against the side of the pool. Spread your arms behind you, hands holding on to the gutter. Lift your left knee, cross it over in front of you, and twist to the right as far as you can. Return to the original position. Lift your right knee, cross it over in front of you, and swing to the left as far as you can. Return to the original position. The water version should be done for thirty seconds every day for two weeks; on the third week, you can increase the time to one minute. The floor version also should be done daily: five times the first week, ten times the second week, fifteen times thereafter, to increase trunk, hip, and knee flexibility and to strengthen abdominal muscles. (F, S)

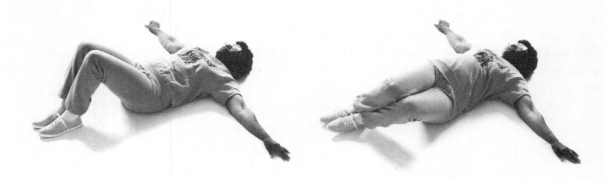

19. Jogging in Place.   Jog in place on a resilient surface, such as a floor mat, or on a treadmill (make sure you hold on). This is best done daily. If a pool is handy, jog at the shallow end, with your arms bent. If it helps, hold on to the side of the pool with one hand. The first week, jog for three minutes; the second week, jog for six minutes; the third week, jog for nine minutes. Breathe deeply to increase your stamina and stimulate your breathing and heartbeat. (CV, S, E)

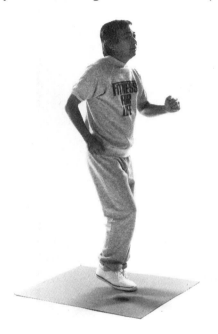

Cool Down Properly!
Finish each exercise session by cooling down. One of the best ways to cool down is to take a five-minute casual walk—no stress, no hurry.

Resist the temptation after exercising to go right into the shower. Rather, you should delay showering until you have stopped sweating. Otherwise, the sweat will keep pouring out after your shower, and you may suffer hypothermia (too rapid loss of body heat) as a result. After your sweating subsides, don a robe or warm-up clothes to prevent the loss of heat.

20. Walking.   This is the wonderful exercise that the human body was designed for. At this level, you should start by walking half a mile at a brisk pace on a smooth, level surface. Swing your arms with enthusiasm, and breathe deeply. If the weather allows, walk outdoors. Dress comfortably and wear a good pair of walking or jogging shoes. If at any time on your walk you feel nauseated or dizzy, stop, sit down, and breathe deeply until you feel better. Walk as often as you can— every other day is best. After a month, you should be able to increase your distance to a mile. This is going to build up your endurance and help your heart and circulatory system as well as tone up your hips, legs, and feet. (CV, E)

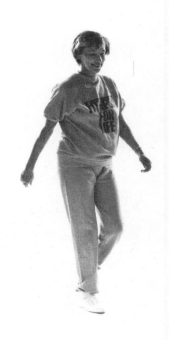

After a month or two at this intensity level, you should be ready to move up to the medium-intensity level, if your fitness goals require additional progress.

12 Exercises at the Medium-Intensity Level

Consider this program of twenty-one exercises if you have kept mildly in shape over the years or if you are now working to get back in shape and have mastered the exercises at the low-medium intensity level.

You've come this far toward the peak of good physical shape as the result of having increased your effort to lift yourself to new heights of fitness. At the summit is your goal: functional fitness.

Even though you may have had friends exercise with you, this is your own accomplishment. No one else could have done it for you. You put out the effort, no one else.

You probably feel better about yourself and your new fitness than you have in a long time. You have a new awareness and confidence in your body. You may view your out-of-shape colleagues and acquaintances who move slowly and with difficulty as "old."

This two-month plan of exercises at a medium level of intensity is characterized by exercises with medium-speed movements that include good doses of mild stress and endurance. The main purpose of this program is to build upon the accomplishments of the previous levels, to provide cardiovascular benefit, to continue increasing the flexibility of your joints, to start emphasizing strengthening of the major muscles, to expand your endurance, and to seriously firm you up.

As at previous levels, you should not experience pain as you go through this plan. However, you should feel some mild muscle soreness the day after you do strength (S) exercises. This is a good indication that you are building strength. You may also experience an unusually relaxed feeling; this is an indication that you are building endurance.

As in the previous chapter, the exercises described here are coded. As you can see, the code refers to fitness goals.

CV = Cardiovascular Fitness
F = Flexibility
S = Strength
E = Endurance
L = Leanness/Slimming
R = Relaxation

Here, as at the lower-level exercise plans, you should do the exercises in the order in which they are presented. These exercises range in difficulty from low-medium to high-medium intensities; begin with smaller muscles and proceed to larger muscles, as in previous chapters; and are the same as some exercises at the low-medium level of intensity.

You should repeat the flexibility and leanness exercises every day, the others at least three times a week.

As at other levels, your medium-level exercise plan will depend on the weather and the availability of facilities and equipment. Three of the exercises can also be done in a swimming pool; an additional three are exclusively for the pool.

The exercises begin at medium levels of intensity (such as ten repetitions) and build up to higher intensity (such as twenty repetitions) and/or to increased loads (weights). Stay with this plan, and after about two months you should be ready for the high-intensity level—if that suits your goals.

The exercises are on the pages that follow.

1. Main Street Stroll and Twist. Simply walk around briskly for six minutes on a level surface. Indoors is OK, but outdoors is even better. Breathe deeply. The first two minutes, walk with an exaggerated swing in your arms, forward and backward. The third and fourth minutes, raise your arms as you walk, and put them through swimming-the-crawl motions. The fifth and sixth minutes, clasp your hands behind your head, and walk with an exaggerated twist of the shoulders—left and then right, and so on. Keep your hips stable in this warm-up exercise that limbers most of your body. It is best if done daily. (F)

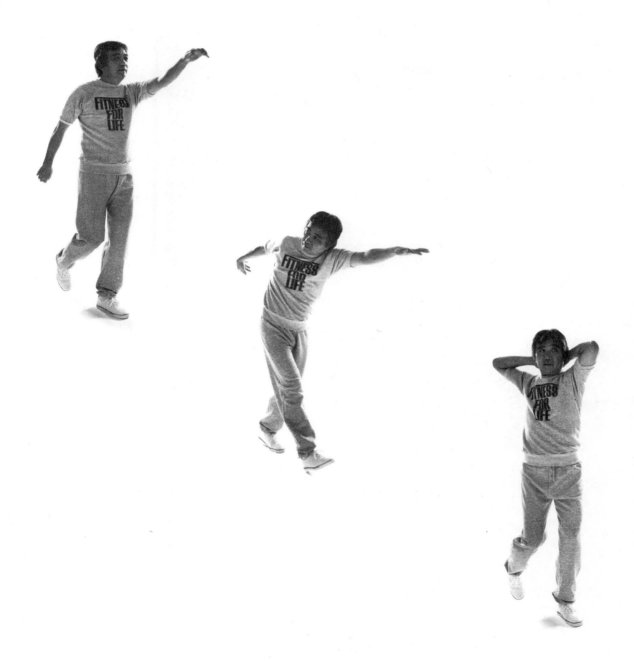

2. Head Roll.   Standing, drop your head back so that you feel the pressure of the muscles back there. Slowly and smoothly, roll your head around in a circle through its entire range of motion. Begin by gently rotating to the left shoulder; then move forward. Keep rotating to the right shoulder, then to the rear again. Close your eyes, and try to relax your shoulders as you revolve your head ten times clockwise and ten times counterclockwise to limber those tight neck muscles and joints. Inhale deeply during half of the revolution; exhale during the

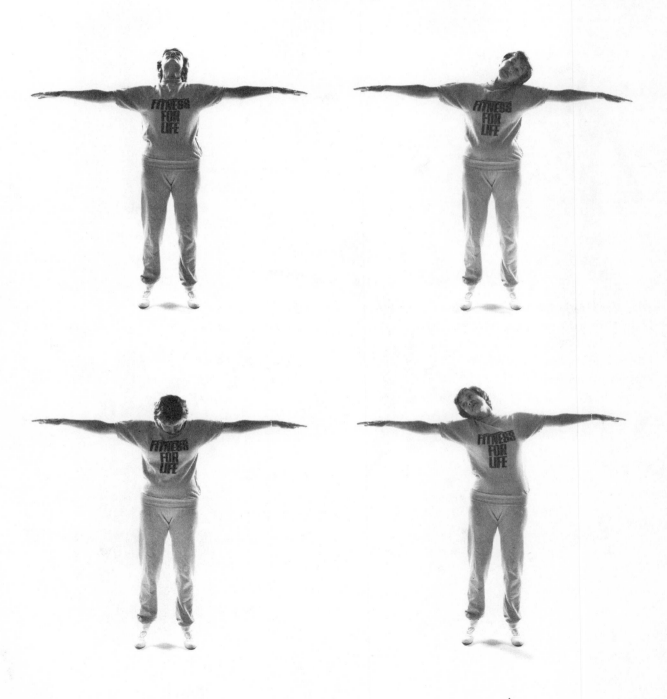

other half. After doing this daily for a month, increase the stretch of the tight muscles by applying a little pressure with your hand at each cardinal point: back (against chin), shoulder (against temple), front (against back of head), shoulder (against temple). (F)

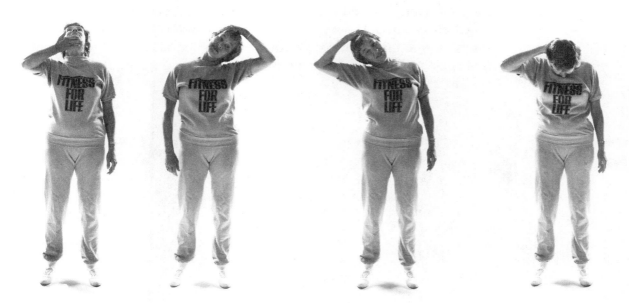

3. Arm Circle. Standing, legs apart, raise both arms at shoulder height to a T position. Make fists with your hands, and tighten the elbows. Then make small circles, keeping your arms rigid. Revolve both arms fifteen times in forward circles, fifteen times in backward circles. Inhale for five circles; exhale for five circles. After that, relax your hands and elbows, and make large circles with your still-extended arms. Revolve fifteen times in big forward circles and fifteen times in big backward circles to limber your shoulders and arms. After doing this daily for a month, hold a can of beans or a book in each hand to build up arm strength and endurance. (F, S)

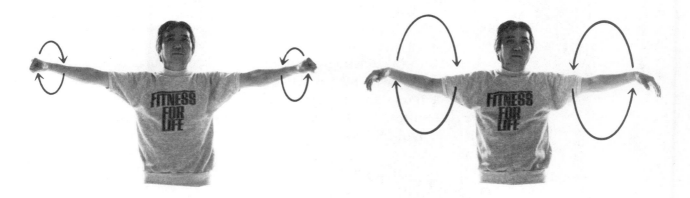

4. Wing Stretcher.   Standing, legs apart, arms straight out to the sides at T position, bend at the elbow to bring your hands to your chest, palms down, with your fingertips touching. This is a four-count exercise. On counts of 1-2-3, pull your elbows back as far as you can. Keep your arms at shoulder height as you pull back three times; then, on count 4, swing your hands all the way, straight out to the sides, turning your palms up. Return to the starting fingertip position. Do this ten times every day for a week. In the second week, increase to twenty times daily to limber and strengthen your upper back, shoulders, arms, and chest and to improve your posture. Exhale on 1-2-3; inhale on 4. (F, S)

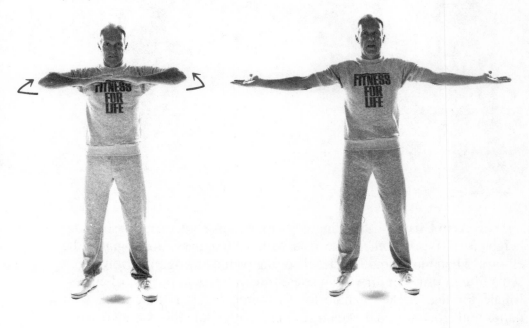

5. Body Side-Bender.   Standing, legs apart, feet spaced as wide as your shoulders, extend your arms straight up, palms facing, fingertips touching. A four-count exercise: (1) bend sideways at the waist to the left as far as you can; (2) return to upright; (3) bend to the right; (4) return to the starting position. Try to keep your elbows straight. Bend smoothly without any jerks, and only as far as you can comfortably. Do ten repetitions every day the first two weeks. The third week, increase to fifteen, and move a little farther with a little more stretch in each bend than you did the first two weeks. The second month, increase to twenty, and try to stretch even a little more yet those arm, leg, and trunk muscles that you are working to limber. Exhale on 1 and 3; inhale on 2 and 4. (F)

6. Flexed-Leg Forward Bend. Standing, feet apart, hold your arms straight over your head, thumbs hooked to each other. Flex (slightly bend) your knees as you bend forward at the waist. Keep the knees bent (to protect your lower back) as you extend your fingertips toward your left toes. Stretch gently. Not touching your toes is all right. Hold it for the count of five. Then stand up. Exhale as you bend; inhale as you rise. Bend forward again, and try to touch your right toes. Do twenty repetitions daily. (F)

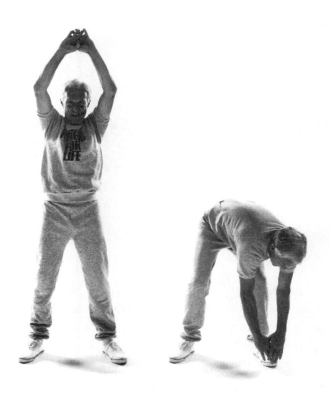

7. Side-Straddle Hop. Also known as a jumping jack, this exercise begins as you stand, feet together, hands hanging down at your sides. The actions of arms and legs are simultaneous in one jumping action. Your legs should be spread widely as your hands come together over your head. Exhale as you do this; then inhale as you jump back to the starting position. Do a daily fifteen vigorously to tone your arms and legs and stimulate your breathing and heart to build endurance. (E)

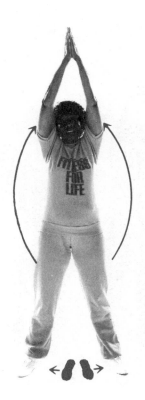

8. Chest Press-Pull.   Standing, feet apart, bring your arms to shoulder height, and bend them at the elbows so that your hands are in front of your chest. Inhale deeply. Exhale as you p-u-s-h your palms against each other. Keep pushing for the count of five. Stop, separate your hands, rotate them in opposite directions, and hook the fingers of one hand to the fingers of the other. Inhale deeply. Exhale as you try to p-u-l-l them apart. Keep pulling for a count of five. Do ten sets of pushes and pulls every other day for the first month, twenty for the second, to strengthen arm, shoulder, and chest muscles. (S)

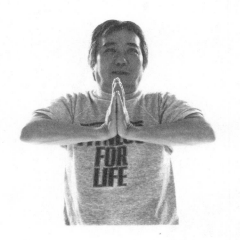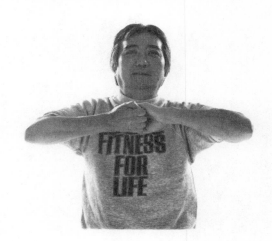

9. Half Knee Bend.   Standing, legs apart, place your hands on your hips. This is a two-count exercise: (1) lower your body a little more than halfway on bent knees as your arms extend forward, palms down; (2) rise, and return to the starting position. Move smoothly, keep your back straight, and breathe deeply. Exhale as you lower your body; inhale as you raise it. Do twelve bends every other day the first month, twenty-five every other day the second month, to strengthen your thigh muscles. (S)

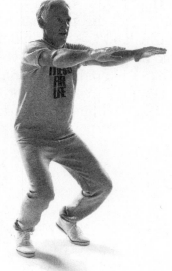

10. Heel Raise. Stand, feet slightly apart, hands at hips, a can of beans or a book in each hand. Raise yourself so that you are standing on your toes; then lower yourself back to the floor. Do this as smoothly as you can. Inhale as you return to starting position; exhale as you raise up. Start with sixteen raises every other day the first month, twenty-five every other day the second, to strengthen your arches, ankles, and calves. For additional strengthening, stand on a book on the floor. Place your weight on the balls of your feet, and keep your heels raised. (S)

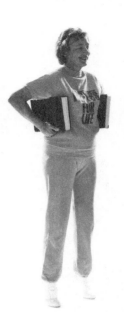

11. Head Curl. Lying on your back on a carpet or mat, stretch out your legs, and hold them together. Cross your arms over your chest. Lift your head and shoulders off the floor. Hold for a count of five. You should feel a good tightness in your abdomen. Lower your head and shoulders, and elbows, to the floor. Breathe deeply. Exhale on rising; inhale on relaxing. Do twenty-five a day of this, the best tummy-firming exercise. (S, L)

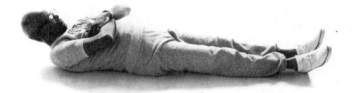

12. Leg Lift. Lying on your back on a carpet or mat, stretch out your legs, and hold them together. Place your hands under your hips, palms down. Raise your left leg, knee straight, off the floor. Hold it for a count of five. Then lower it back to the floor. Inhale deeply. Exhale as you raise the straightened right leg and hold for a count of five. Repeat fifteen times to strengthen the abdominal and front thigh muscles. After doing this every other day for a month, try holding each leg up for a count of ten. (Do *not* try this with both legs at once, as this will place too much stress on the lower back.) (S)

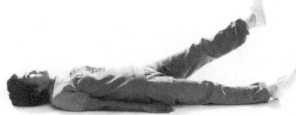

13. Side Leg Raise.   Lying on your right side on a carpet or mat, extend your straightened right arm in line with your body. Rest your head on the arm. Your left arm in front of you, palm on floor, helps balance you. Start with your legs together. Smoothly raise the straightened left leg as high as you can (vertical is ideal). Slowly lower it back to its original position. Do this fifteen times. Then roll over to your left side, and raise the right leg fifteen times. Do each leg five times again. Done daily, this exercise strengthens hip and outer thigh muscles and firms up those "love handles" on your flanks. Exhale as you raise each leg; inhale as you lower the leg. (S, L)

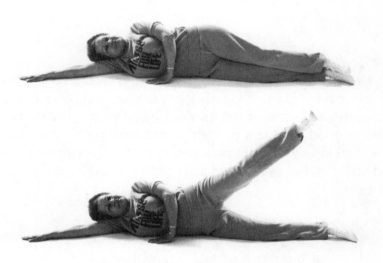

14. Knee Push-up.   Lying on your tummy, legs together, place your hands under your shoulders, palms on the floor. Bend your knees so as to raise your feet off the floor. Now, keeping your back straight, push against the floor until your arms are fully extended and your body, from the knees up, is off the floor. Slowly lower yourself to the floor, keeping your knees bent. Do fifteen this month, twenty-five next month. Done every other day, this strengthens arm, shoulder, chest, and abdominal muscles. (S)

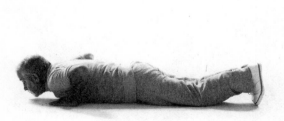 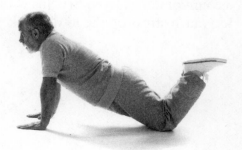

15. Flutter Kick.   On the floor, lie facedown, and tuck your hands under your thighs. Arch your back so as to bring your head off the floor and your legs off the floor, toes pointed. Hold this position as you slightly separate your legs and kick them in a continuous flutter for a minute. Next month, increase the time to two minutes. The legs should kick from the hip, with the knees only slightly bent. This can also be done in a swimming pool. Lie on your front, and hold on to the side of the pool. Point your toes, and kick in a whip action with knees and ankles flexible. Do a minute daily now and two minutes daily in a month to limber and strengthen your back, your buttocks, and the back of your neck and thighs. (F, S)

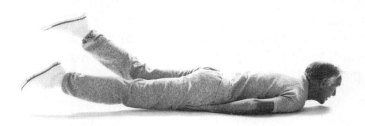

16. Raised-Knee Crossover.   Lie on your back, arms spread-eagle. Raise both knees together until your thighs are vertical; then swing them to the left as far as you can, trying to touch your knees to the floor. Then swing back to the center, and twist to the right as far as you can. Exhale deeply as you twist to the side; inhale as you return to the center position. This can also be done in a pool. Stand in chest-deep water with your back against the side of the pool. Spread your arms behind you, hands holding on to the gutter. Lift your left knee, cross it over in front of you, and twist to the right as far as you can. Return to the original position. Lift your right knee, cross it over in front of you, and swing to the left as far as you can. Return to the original position. Daily do twenty-five repetitions of the floor version or three minutes of the water version to increase trunk, hip, and knee flexibility and to strengthen abdominal muscles. (F, S)

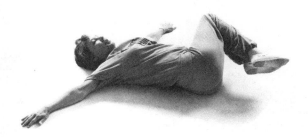

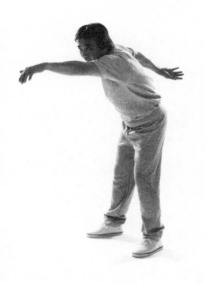

17. Standing Crawl. Standing, bend forward and move your arms through the crawl stroke actions. (Make sure your legs are firmly planted on the floor so you can maintain your balance.) Reach out with your left hand and dip into the "water." Get a "grip" on the "water," press downward, and pull your hand back. Keep pulling your hand past your body as far as you can. As your left hand comes by the left side, your right hand should reach out. Keep the left and right hands working in a rhythm of opposition. Rotate your head as you "swim" so that as your left hand goes into the "water," your head turns to the right and you inhale. As your left hand comes back and your right hand goes out, your head should rotate to the left. When your face is straight down, forcefully exhale. "Swim" like this for five minutes. In a swimming pool, stand in chest-deep water, and place each foot behind you on the edge of the pool. Move your arms to keep your head up as you do the crawl stroke, pulling each hand past your thigh and out of the water. On land or in the water, do this every day to limber your arms, shoulders, and upper back. (F, L)

18. Walking-Jogging.   At this level, you should start by walking a mile at a brisk pace on a smooth, level surface. Swing your arms with enthusiasm, and breathe deeply. If the weather allows, walk outdoors. Other times, use an indoor track or a treadmill. Dress comfortably, and wear a good pair of jogging shoes. Walk as often as you can—every other day is best. After two weeks, walk two miles. After a month, start jogging ten steps to every fifty you walk. This "interval training" is going to build up your endurance and help your heart and circulatory system, as well as tone up your hips, legs, and feet. (CV, E)

Cooling Down

Finish each exercise session by cooling down.

One of the best ways to cool down is to take a five-minute casual walk—no stress, no hurry.

Resist the temptation after exercising to go right into the shower. Rather, you should delay showering until you have stopped sweating. Otherwise, the sweat will keep pouring out after your shower, and you may suffer hypothermia (too-rapid loss of body heat) as a result. After your sweating subsides, don a robe or warm-up clothes to prevent the loss of heat.

When you sweat, you lose a lot of water, so drink orange juice or tomato juice to replace your fluids and minerals.

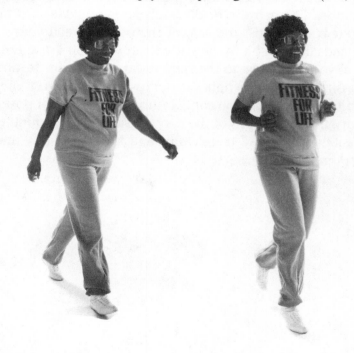

The following three exercises are exclusively for the pool.

19. Bobs.   In the pool, in chest-high water, take a deep breath, hold it, and submerge as you bend your knees. Exhale as you descend. Push yourself up to the standing position, and inhale. Do as many as you can in a minute. Repeat every day. After two weeks, increase the bobbing period to two minutes and after three weeks to three minutes to advance your endurance. (E)

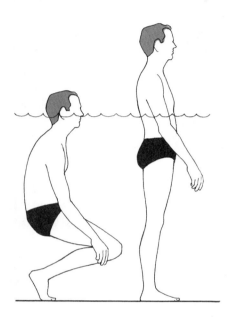

20. Treading.   This must be done at the deep end of the pool, where your feet cannot touch bottom. Simply move your feet so as to keep your head above water. Use the bicycle, scissors, or frog kick. Use your arms to stabilize yourself and to keep vertical. At first, tread water for a minute. Breath control is a must in this exercise, which is best done every day or every other day. After two weeks, increase your time to two minutes. Over the two months, try to build up to five minutes to strengthen your legs and lower abdominal muscles and to increase your endurance. (S, E)

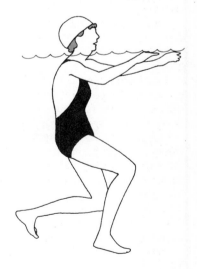

21. Swimming Crawl. Put your flutter kick and your crawl stroke together and swim laps of the pool for five minutes. See how many lengths you can build up to in the next two months. Try to increase your endurance so that you are swimming fifteen and twenty minutes at a time three times a week. As an exercise, swimming is wonderful for limbering your arms, shoulders, trunk, and legs; for slimming; for improving endurance; for cardiovascular fitness; and for improving coordination. Furthermore, after a good swim, you will feel very relaxed. (CV, F, E, L, R)

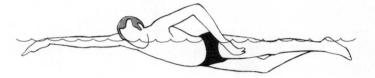

After two months at this medium-intensity level, you should be ready to move up to the high-intensity level, if your fitness goals require additional progress.

13 Exercises at the High-Intensity Level

As one who enjoys life, including leisure, as much as anyone, I maintain exercise is one essential that not only helps you enjoy the life you have, but can help you have more life to enjoy.
—Kenneth H. Cooper, Aerobic Center, Dallas

Consider this plan of thirty-three exercises if you are in good shape and/or have mastered the exercises at the medium level of intensity.

You have lifted yourself to new heights of fitness by reaching this plateau. Ahead is the summit and your goal: functional fitness.

You have now succeeded in matching, or exceeding, the fitness level of your youth. Then fitness was not as important to function as it is at this age. Now you can achieve the maximum fitness possible by following this three-month plan of exercises at the high-intensity level.

This plan is characterized by exercises that require medium to high effort and medium to fast movements that include stress and endurance as major components. The main purpose of this plan is to build upon the accomplishments of the previous levels, to continue increasing the flexibility of your joints, to give your body new firmness and leanness, to increase the strength of major muscles, to provide maximum cardiovascular benefit, and to expand your endurance to the limit.

As at previous levels, you should not experience pain as you go through this exercise plan. However, you will feel some mild muscle soreness the day after you do strength exercises. This is a good indication that you are building strength.

Not long after each workout, you will also experience an unusually relaxed feeling, an indication that you are building endurance. That is a very good time to practice your relaxation technique. These combined abilities to relax will allow you to sleep better than you ever have before. (See chapter 8.)

As in the previous chapters, the exercises described here are coded according to fitness goals.

CV = Cardiovascular Fitness
F = Flexibility
S = Strength
E = Endurance
L = Leanness/Slimming
R = Relaxation

Here, as at the lower-level exercise plans, you should do the flexibility and strength exercises in the order in which they are presented. Some of the exercises here are the same as those at the medium level. In addition, there are eleven endurance activities here to choose from. Five of the exercises are designed for use in a swimming pool.

You should repeat the flexibility and leanness exercises that are in your program every day, the other exercises in your program at least three times a week. *Always* do the flexibility exercises before *and* after your endurance exercising as a way of warming up and cooling down.

The exercises begin at medium levels of intensity (such as ten repetitions) and build up to high intensity (such as twenty repetitions) and/or to increased loads (weights) and endurance levels. Stay with this plan, and after about three months, you should be at the peak—if that suits your goals. If you want to stay at the peak, or at any plateau, you must keep up your exercise program. If you do not, you will slide back to a lower plateau and, eventually, to the Valley of Unfitness below.

This peak called Endurance can be defined as the ability to *not* get out of breath right away. When you start your endurance exercises, you will notice that you quickly run out of breath. But the more you do them and the more you extend yourself, the longer you will be able to go before you get out of breath. That's what endurance is all about.

Your achievement of higher and higher stages of endurance means that your body has achieved higher and higher levels of aerobic capacity, the ability to use oxygen. You will be surprised by two wonderful new feelings when you swim, run, cycle, jump rope, or whatever.

One is deeper, slower breathing. This indicates that you are using oxygen in ways your body never did before or hasn't done in many years.

The other wonderful new feeling is your slow heartbeat. You are able to exert yourself for extended periods of time without your heart beating so fast it feels as if it is in your throat. That's because your heart has become far more efficient with every beat than it was before you were in shape.

Both of these new feelings mean that you have achieved new levels of inner equilibrium in high-intensity activities.

That's endurance!

While these endurance activities will automatically force you to breathe deeply, other exercises, particularly those at the beginning of your daily routine, will not. When you do these exercises, you have to consciously breathe deeply.

Note that the first twelve exercises are flexibility exercises that you should consider also as warm-up exercises to do before endurance exercises. The next ten are strengthening exercises. The final eleven are endurance exercises. At this level, probably having been involved in fitness for several months, you might have some favorite exercises of your own that enhance flexibility and build muscle strength and endurance. By all means, substitute them for the ones here in any of the three categories. After all, this is *your* program, and you have to be comfortable with it if you are going to stay on it.

The exercises are on the pages that follow.

A Dozen for Flexibility

1. Main Street Stroll and Twist.   Simply walk around briskly for six minutes on a level surface. Indoors is OK, but outdoors is even better. Breathe deeply. The first two minutes, walk with an exaggerated forward and backward swing in your arms. The third and fourth minutes, raise your arms as you walk, and put them through swimming-the-crawl motions. The fifth and sixth minutes, clasp your hands behind your head, and walk with an exaggerated twist of the shoulders—left and then right, and so on. Keep your hips stable in this warm-up exercise that limbers most of your body. For cooling down, do three minutes. (F)

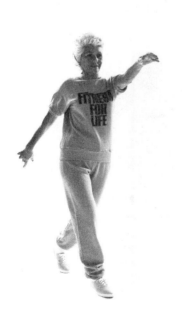
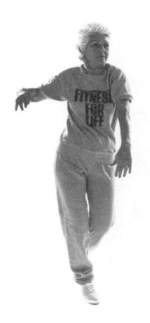
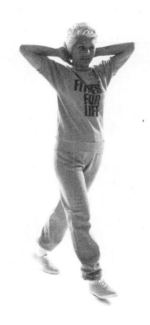

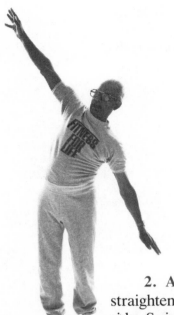

2. Arm Propeller.   Standing, legs slightly apart, raise your straightened right arm above your head; let the left arm drop to your side. Swing your arms simultaneously in big circles, like airplane propellers, always opposite each other. Breathe deeply in rhythm with the rotations. Do fifteen seconds, or fifteen circles, in one direction and then fifteen seconds or circles in the opposite direction to loosen up your shoulders, elbows, and wrists. For cool-down, do half as many. (F)

3. Wing Stretcher.   Standing, legs apart, arms straight out to the sides at T position, bend at the elbow to bring your hands to your chest, palms down, with your fingertips touching. This is a four-count exercise. On each count of 1-2-3, pull your elbows back as far as you can. Keep your arms at shoulder height as you pull back three times; then, on count 4, swing your hands all the way, straight out to the sides,

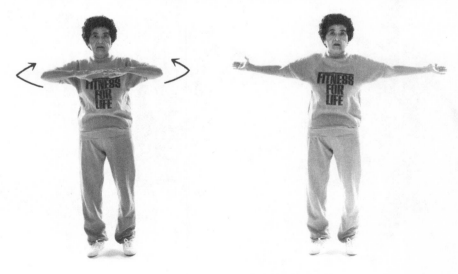

turning your palms up. Return to the starting fingertip position. Inhale on the flyback; exhale when you bring your arms forward. Do this twenty times every day to limber and strengthen your upper back, shoulders, arms, and chest and to improve your posture. Do half as many for cool-down. (F, S)

4. Body Side-Bender. Stand, legs apart, feet spaced as wide as your shoulders, hands interlaced behind your neck. A four-count exercise: (1) bend sideways at the waist to the left as far as you can; (2) return to an upright position; (3) bend to the right; (4) return to the starting position. Try to keep your elbows straight. Bend smoothly without any jerks, but try to s-t-r-e-t-c-h those trunk muscles. Feel the stretch, but not to the point of pain. Exhale on the stretch; inhale on the return. Do ten repetitions every day. Do five for cool-down. (F)

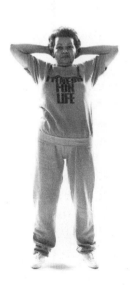
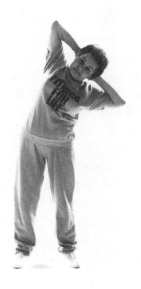

5. Alternate Floor Touch. Stand, legs far apart, arms out at shoulder height in a T position. A four-count exercise: (1) bend forward at the waist as you rotate your trunk to position your right hand (arms still straight) to touch your left toes; (2) return to a standing position; (3) bend down, this time rotating your body so that your left hand touches your right toes; (4) stand straight. Do ten times to limber your arms, back, and trunk and the backs of your legs. Exhale on the stretch; inhale on the return. Do five times for cool-down. (This exercise is most effective when you keep the knees straight; but if you have a lower-back problem, bending the knees a bit is OK. Not quite touching your toes is OK, too.) (F)

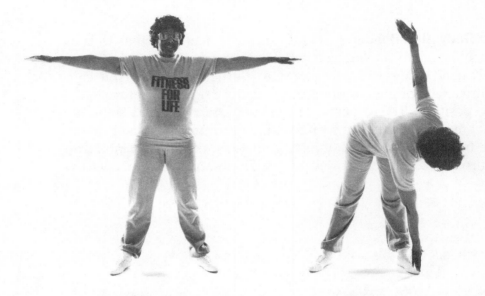

6. Sitting Stretch. Sitting on the floor, back straight, legs straight and spread in front of you, hands resting on knees, bend forward from the waist. Extend your hands as far forward as you can. If you can touch your ankles, fine; if you can touch your toes, better; if you can touch the floor beyond your toes, best. Feel the s-t-r-e-t-c-h, but not to the point of pain. Hold it for five seconds; then return to the sitting position. Every day try to stretch a little beyond the previous day's limit. Exhale on the stretch; inhale on the return. Do ten to stretch the muscles of your arms, back, and the backs of your legs. Do five for cool-down. (F)

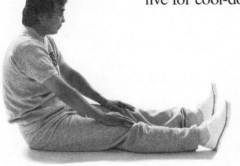
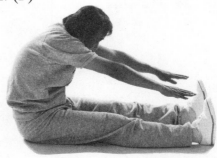

7. Head Curl.   Lying on your back, stretch out your legs, and hold them together. Clasp your hands behind your neck. Lift your head and shoulders off the floor in a curling motion with your chin tucked in, your shoulders and back rounded. Hold it for a count of ten. You should feel a good tightness in your abdomen. Lower your head and shoulders, and elbows, to the floor. Breathe deeply. Exhale on rising; inhale on relaxing. Do twenty-five a day to stretch your back and firm your tummy. Do ten for cool-down. (F, S, L)

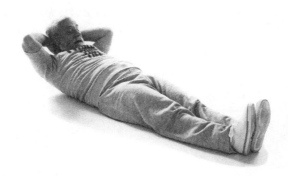

8. Side Leg Raise and Whip.   Lying on your right side, extend your straightened right arm in line with your body. Rest your head on the arm. Your left arm in front of your chest, palm on the floor, helps balance you. Start with your legs together. Smoothly but quickly raise the straightened left leg as high as you can (vertical is ideal). Slowly lower it back to its original position. Do this ten times. Then roll over to your left side and raise the right leg ten times. Do five of each leg for cool-down. Once you feel you have mastered the *leg raise,* try the *leg whip:* whip each leg up and down as high and as fast as you can. This takes strength and flexibility. Done daily, both raises and whips increase flexibility of the hips; strengthen trunk, hip, and outer thigh muscles; and firm up "love handles." (F, S, L)

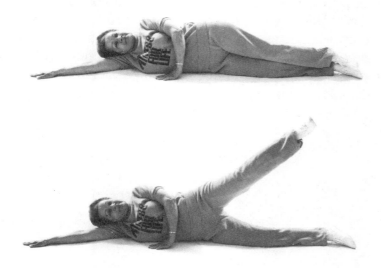

9. Leg Stretch.   Lying on your back, bend your knees, keeping your feet on the floor. Place your hands at your sides. Raise your right leg toward the ceiling, and try to straighten your knee. Do not jerk or bounce it. Hold it for a count of five. Then lower it back to the original position. Inhale deeply. Exhale as you raise the left leg, and hold it up for a count of five. If you want more of a stretch, push your heel up toward the ceiling. Repeat ten times to stretch the hamstring muscles and the Achilles tendon and to strengthen the abdominal and front thigh muscles. Do five for cool-down. After doing this for a month, try holding each leg up for a count of ten. (Do *not* try this with both legs at once, since this will place too much stress on your lower back.) (F, S)

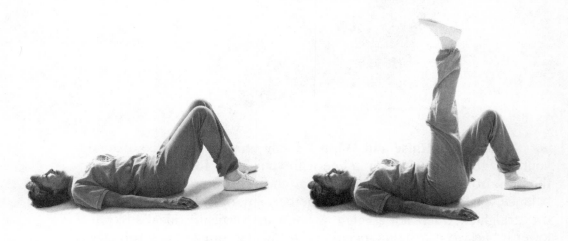

10. Knee Raise and Hug.   Lying on your back, legs extended, feet together, arms at sides, raise your left leg about a foot off the floor. Hold it for a count of five; then bend the knee and pull it toward your chest. Clasp the knee with both hands, and pull it gently toward your chest as far as possible. Count to five; then return the knee to its original position. Exhale as you lift the leg and knee; inhale as you lower them. Then do the right leg and knee. Do ten to improve the flexibility of your knees and hip joints and to strengthen your abdominal muscles. Do five for cool-down. (F, S)

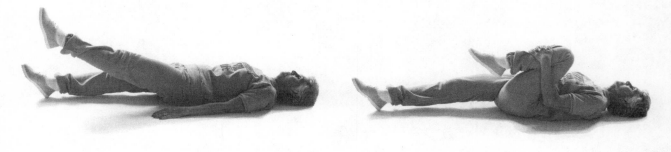

11. Flutter Kick.   On the floor, lie facedown, and tuck your hands under your thighs. Arch your back so as to bring your head off the floor and your legs off the floor, toes pointed. Hold this position as you slightly separate your legs and kick them in a continuous flutter for a minute. The legs should kick from the hips, with the knees only slightly bent. This can also be done in the swimming pool. Lie on your front, and hold on to the side of the pool. Point your toes, and kick in a whip action, with knees and ankles flexible, for a minute to limber and strengthen your back, your buttocks, the back of your neck, and the backs of your thighs. For cooling down, do half a minute. (F, S)

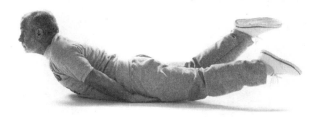

12. Sprinter.   Assume the sprinter's starting position—both hands on the floor, fingers extended forward bearing most of your weight, right leg in squat position curled under you, left leg fully extended to the rear. This is a two-count exercise: (1) In a bouncing movement, reverse the position of the feet; bring the left foot to the left hand, extending the right foot all the way to the rear. Hold for a count of three as you stretch the right leg. Inhale. (2) Reverse the feet to the starting position. Hold for a count of three as you stretch the left leg. Exhale. The first times you do this, stretch gently so as not to hurt anything. As your flexibility improves, you can increase the stretch tension. Do five times daily to tone and stretch the muscles and tendons of the backs of the legs (which are heavily used in walking, jogging, bicycling, and swimming). After two weeks increase to ten times after a month to fifteen, and after two months to twenty. For cooling down, do five. (F)

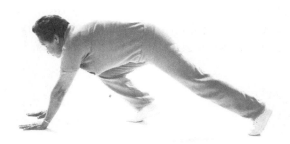

Ten for Strength

13. Chest Press-Pull. Standing, feet apart, bring your arms to shoulder height, and bend them at the elbows so that your hands are in front of your chest. Inhale deeply. Exhale as you p-u-s-h your palms against each other. Keep pushing for the count of five. Stop, and separate your hands; then rotate them in opposite directions, and hook the fingers of one hand to those of the other. Inhale deeply. Exhale as you try to p-u-l-l the fingers apart. Keep pulling for a count of five. Do twenty sets of pushes and pulls every other day to strengthen arm, shoulder, and chest muscles. (S)

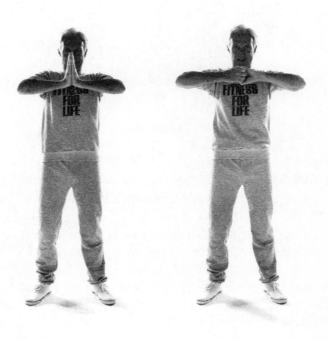

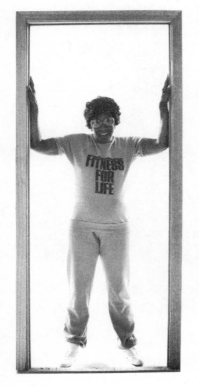

14. Samson Door Press. Stand in an open doorway with your feet apart. Lift your bent arms to about shoulder height (if the door opening allows), and place your hands on opposite jambs of the door frame. Push out a la Samson pushing over the pillars in ancient Israel. Exhale as you push. Hold for a count of ten. Relax, and inhale. Repeat ten times to build strength in your upper arms, shoulders, and upper back. (S)

15. Arm Curl. In each hand, hold an object that weighs two to three pounds, such as a can of beans, a book, or a dumbbell. Both hands should be hanging at your sides. Bend the right arm as you lift the weight as high as you can—to your shoulder, if possible. Exhale with this action. Lower the right hand as you raise the left; inhale. Do ten curls for each arm. After a month, change the weight to five pounds, and work up to fifteen curls. After two months, go to ten pounds to strengthen your upper arms and hands. (S)

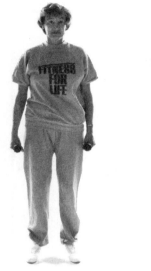
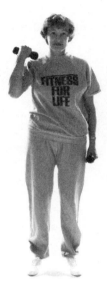

16. Arm Extension. In your left hand, hold an object that weighs two to three pounds, such as a two-pound or three-pound can of coffee (in a plastic bag if your hands are small), a book, or a dumbbell. Lift that hand and weight overhead; then slowly bend your arm until the hand holding the weight is behind your head. Slowly lift the weight until your arm is fully extended. Do ten times; then switch the weight to the right hand and do ten with that arm. After a month, go to five pounds, and work up to fifteen repetitions. After two months, go to ten pounds to strengthen your shoulders, upper arms, and hands. (S)

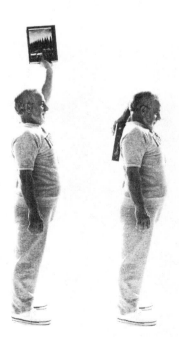

17. Chest Fly.   With a book, can, or small dumbbell weighing two or three pounds in each hand, lie on your back on a bench or on the floor, knees bent. Hold your arms straight above your chest, and inhale deeply as you spread your arms to the sides with your elbows slightly bent. Exhale forcefully as you bring your arms (and weights) back to their starting position above your chest. At each session every other day, do five times the first two weeks, ten times for the third and fourth weeks, and fifteen times for the fifth and sixth weeks. On the seventh week, increase the weight to five pounds, and start the same cycle of five, ten, and fifteen repetitions for the seventh and eighth, ninth and tenth, and eleventh and twelfth weeks, to strengthen your chest muscles and improve shoulder motion in the lateral direction. (S)

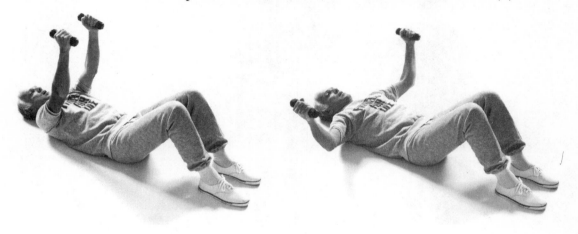

18. Squat.   Standing, legs slightly apart, extend your arms straight ahead of you. This is a two-count exercise: (1) exhale as you lower your body to a nearly sitting position so that your thighs are parallel to the floor or until your buttocks just about touch the seat of a

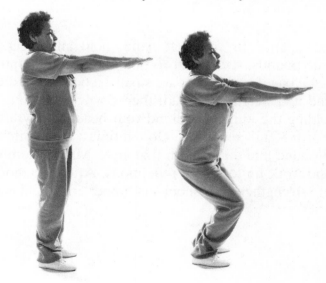

chair; (2) inhale as you *slowly* rise and return to the standing position. Move smoothly, keep your back straight, and breathe deeply. Do six squats every other day the first month, twelve every other day the second month, and twenty every other day the third month, to strengthen your thigh muscles. (S)

19. Heel Raise. Stand, feet slightly apart, hands at sides, a five-pound dumbbell in each hand. Raise yourself so that you are standing on your toes; then lower yourself back to the floor. Do this as smoothly as you can. Inhale as you return to the starting position; exhale as you raise yourself up. Do ten raises every other day the first month, twenty every other day the second, and thirty every other day the third, to strengthen your arches, ankles, and calves. For additional strengthening, stand on a book on the floor. Place your weight on the balls of your feet, and keep your heels raised. (S)

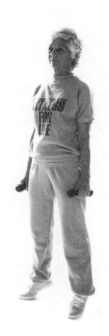

20. Sit-up. Lie on your back, hands folded behind your head, knees bent, feet on the floor. Have someone sit on your feet, or hook your feet under a heavy piece of furniture. Exhale as you curl your body upward. As you reach the sitting position, twist your body so that your right elbow touches your left knee (or comes close to it). The next time up, touch your left elbow to your right knee. Keep your lower back as straight as possible. Every other day during the first month, do ten, the second month twenty-five, the third month forty, to strengthen your abdominal muscles. (S)

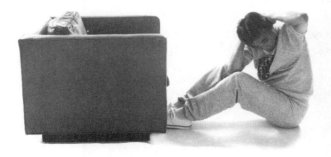

21. Push-up.   Lying on the floor, facedown, place your hands under your shoulders, palms on the floor, fingers pointing straight ahead. Your legs should be together, toes touching the floor. Now, take a deep breath, and, keeping your back straight, push until your body is raised to the height of your fully extended arms. Exhale forcefully as you push. All of your weight should rest on your hands and toes. Slowly lower yourself until your chest touches the floor, keeping your knees and back straight and your buttocks in line with the rest of your body. Inhale as you lower yourself. Do, every other day, five per set this month, twelve per set next month, and twenty-five per set the third month, to strengthen arm, shoulder, chest, and abdominal muscles. (If you have high blood pressure, this exercise is not for you.) (S)

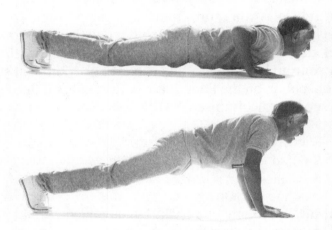

22. Raised-Knee Crossover.   Lie on your back, arms spread-eagle. Raise both knees together until your thighs are vertical; then swing your knees smoothly to the left as far as you can, trying to touch them to the floor. Swing back to the center, and smoothly twist to the right as far as you can. Finally, return to the center, and straighten your legs. Exhale deeply as you twist to the side; inhale as you return to the center position. This can be done twenty times daily this month, thirty times daily next month, and forty times daily the third month, to increase trunk, hip, and knee flexibility and to strengthen leg and abdominal muscles. (This can also be done in water, with your arms along the sides of the pool behind you.) (F, S)

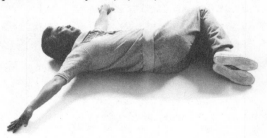

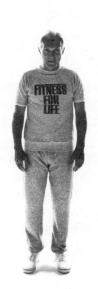
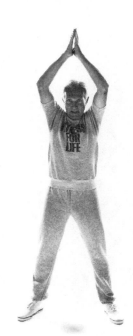

Eight on Dry Land for Cardiovascular Fitness and Endurance

23. Side-Straddle Hop. This exercise, also known as a jumping jack, is a good one for getting ready for endurance activities. You begin by standing, feet together, hands hanging down at your sides. The actions of arms and legs are simultaneous in one jumping action—legs spread widely as hands come together over the head. Exhale as you do this; then inhale as you jump back to the starting position. Do a daily twenty vigorously to tone your arms and legs and stimulate your breathing and heart to build endurance. (E)

24. Stair Climbing. The nice thing about stairs is that there are plenty of them around, they are free equipment, and weather is never a problem. Stairs, plus two good legs, are all you need (although skilled amputees accomplish this, too). Start out with a small dose because you will feel fine with the first steps but will very quickly tire out. Climb and descend for a total of five minutes at first. Breathe deeply, and follow this five-point plan: (1) climb two flights, (2) walk around, (3) climb two flights, (4) walk around, and (5) descend. Do this three times a week for a month, and then increase your time to seven and a half minutes. Go to ten minutes three times a week at the start of the third month. After ninety days, you should be ready for fifteen minutes three times a week. Climbing stairs exercises the muscles at the front of the thighs, and descending uses the muscles at the back of the thighs. (This is not recommended for persons who have not kept in shape for years or who have balance problems.) (CV, E)

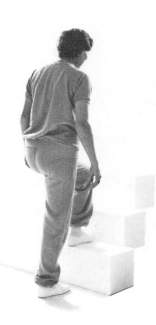

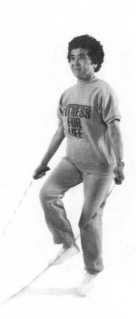

25. Rope Skipping.   Like stair climbing, this is a convenient, weatherproof exercise. In rope skipping, you follow the principles of interval training: you skip for a certain period of time, then rest, then resume skipping, and so on. Start by skipping for fifteen seconds, then resting for thirty seconds. Try to total three minutes of skipping time (do not include resting time). That would be twelve sets. Breathe deeply, and repeat three times a week. In the second month, you should be doing twenty sets of thirty-second skipping with thirty-second rests, for a total skipping time of ten minutes, three times a week. In the third month, you should be doing twenty sets of one-minute skipping with thirty-second rests, for a total of twenty minutes, three times a week. Before you start skipping rope, make sure your calves are strong (the heel raise is a great conditioner of calf muscles). (This is not recommended for anyone with a balance problem or anyone who has not been in shape for years.) (CV, E)

26. Dancing.   Active, vigorous dancing, including square dancing and the commercial exercise dances (Aerobic Dance and Jazzercise), is a very good form of exercise for endurance and your heart. It is good if you maintain it for twenty minutes or more and are sweating by the time you are done. Make sure your dance leader is knowledgeable and experienced; then you'll have some assurance that your movements are appropriate for your level of fitness and skill. Also, you should be dancing like this three times a week if you choose this form of exercise. (CV, E)

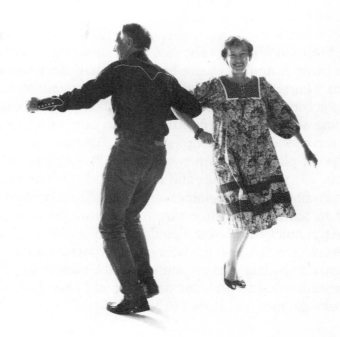

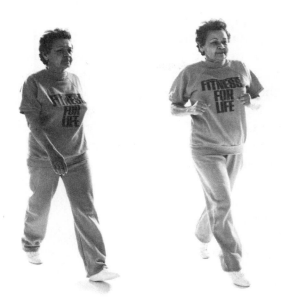

27. Walking-Jogging. At this level, you should start increasing your brisk walking, walking-jogging, or jogging to a goal of three miles three or four times a week. You should do a mile the first month, increase to two miles the next month, and increase to three miles the third month. Walk at a brisk pace on a smooth, level surface. Swing your arms with enthusiasm, and breathe deeply. To walk-jog, work up to alternating walking with jogging. If you have never jogged before, don't start now without your doctor's approval; walk instead. But if you do jog, work up your speed as well as your distance. Jog every other day to allow your feet, knees, and hips to recover. When the weather allows, go outdoors. Other times, use an indoor track, treadmill, or minitrampoline. Dress comfortably, and wear a good pair of jogging shoes. Wear a radio headset if you wish, but don't let it reduce your alertness to traffic, dogs, and other hazards. Remember, while this helps your heart and circulatory system, it is *not* a well-rounded exercise. It is terrific for exercising your hips, the backs of your legs, and your feet, but it does nothing for the front part of your legs or for your upper body, so complement this with another activity for well-roundedness. (CV, E)

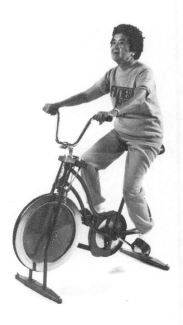

28. Cycling. If you were an active bicycler any previous time in your life, you might want to consider taking cycling up again as an endurance activity. A few turns around the block and you'll feel those old skills sharpening again. But if you never learned to ride a bike, this is not the time to start unless you know that your balance is perfect. Indoor stationary cycling is something else; it is safe and stable, and no balance ability is required. Whichever form fits you, pedaling is a very good way to build up endurance and to get cardiovascular exercise. Start out by doing a mile three times a week. After two weeks, go up to two miles three times a week. Increase one mile every two weeks until, at the end of three months, you are pedaling six-mile distances. Also work to increase your speed. If you bicycle outside, be sure to wear a helmet and observe safety precautions and all traffic rules. Motorists show little regard for those millions of bicycles on streets and roads. Stationary cycling is apt to be boring, but you can spend this half hour reading a book, watching TV, or listening to stereo. (CV, E)

29. Nordic, or Cross-Country, Skiing. Cross-country (or X-C) skiing is one of the most vigorous activities you can undertake. You can do it outdoors in the winter or indoors on special equipment any time of the year. Don't start outdoor skiing if you have never skied before unless you have perfect balance. But if you have skied before, even if only downhill (Alpine), you might want to consider this version. You do need snow, but you can ski on any level surface—a park or a field will do as well as a national forest. The first few times, go with someone who knows the sport and can teach you. Try a half hour to start, and build up to an hour or more. Dress in layers so that you are not too cold when you begin or too warm when you finish. As for the indoor X-C equipment, a half hour is a good goal. Cross-country skiing builds up not only endurance but also your arms and legs. (CV, S, E)

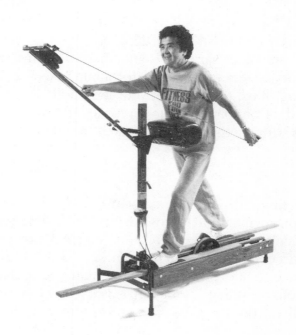

30. Rowing. While this is vigorous enough an exercise to build endurance, it stresses only the arms and shoulders. Thus it is far from well rounded as an activity and, furthermore, can be a problem for persons with high blood pressure. If done outside, it is seasonally limited to summer. If an indoor rowing machine workout makes you sweat for twenty minutes or so, and you happen to like it, fine. (CV, S, E)

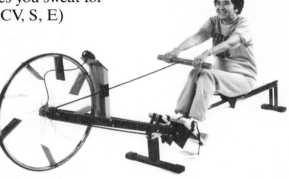

Three in the Pool for Cardiovascular Fitness and Endurance

31. High Bobbing. In the pool, in water three feet over your head, take a deep breath, hold it, and submerge as you bend your knees and extend your arms up. Exhale as you descend. At the end of your downward motion, bring your arms to your sides, and bring the legs together in a frog kick to push yourself up to the surface. Inhale. Do it again; this time lower yourself to the bottom and jump up, using your arms in a breast stroke to lift your head and shoulders high out of the water. Continue to use the second version, pushing off the bottom of the pool. Do as many as you can in a minute for a total of three minutes. Do this every other day. In the second month, do it for six minutes, every other day, and in the third month, do it for twelve minutes every other day, to advance your endurance. (CV, E)

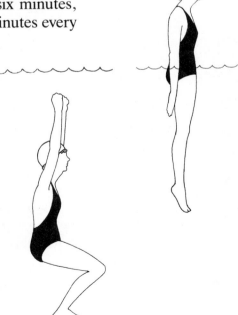

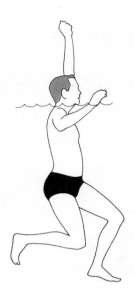

32. Advanced Treading.   This must be done at the deep end of the pool, where your feet cannot touch bottom. Move your feet so as to keep your head above water. Use the bicycle, scissors, or frog kick. Keep one arm out of the water, held high. Breath control is a must in this exercise, which is best done every day or every other day. At first, tread water for a minute. After two weeks, increase your time to two minutes. By the end of the first month, build up to three minutes. In the second month, build up to five minutes, and try keeping both arms high out of the water. In the third month, do ten minutes with both arms out to strengthen your legs and lower abdomen and to increase your endurance. (CV, S, E)

33. Lap Swimming.   Using the crawl, swim as many lengths of the pool as you can before getting winded. Ease off by using a lazy breaststroke or sidestroke until you feel recovered; then resume with the crawl. You should be swimming for twenty minutes or more. Find out how many laps of the pool it takes to cover a quarter of a mile, half a mile, and a full mile, and use those as goals. By the end of three months, you should be doing a mile. A technique that competitive swimmers use is interval training. You swim hard for four lengths, then easy for four, then hard for four, and so on, alternating for the full distance of your workout. As an exercise, swimming is wonderful for limbering your arms, shoulders, trunk, and legs; for slimming; for improving endurance; for cardiovascular fitness; and for improving coordination. Furthermore, after a good swim, you will feel very relaxed. (CV, F, E, L, R)

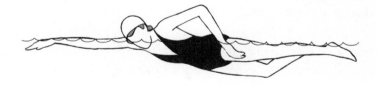

After three months at this high-intensity level, you should be ready to do anything! Once you are at the peak, you have to work to stay there. Keep up your exercise program. You now may want to consider some sports. (See chapter 16.)

14 Pain, Injury, Illness—Prevention and Treatment

"No one should have pain," says a well-known trainer who has worked with thousands of older persons. "Pain is the body's warning system. One must find out the 'why' of pain. For over 50 percent of senior citizens, pain is due to weakness and tightness."

The observation is that of Robert R. Spackman, Jr., head sports trainer at Southern Illinois University, Carbondale, for twenty-three years and now trainer-therapist at S.I.U.'s Wellness Center.

"Doc" Spackman believes, "We don't stop exercising because we are old—we get old because we stop exercising." Limbs that are unused grow soft outside and tight inside. Accompanying the softness and tightness are the limitations of joint movement that come in small increments over the years. Some, not all, of these limitations may be due to arthritis. Together, these conditions set up an increased risk of injury, strains, and sprains, all of which announce their presence by pain. (That's pain as distinguished from muscular aches, which often occur when you start exercising muscles that haven't been exercised in years.) That is why, after the medical considerations discussed in an earlier chapter, prevention of pain and injury is a foremost consideration in putting together a program of exercise for middle-aged and older adults.

Rhythmic exercises and sports involve the repetitive action of groups of large muscles, especially in the legs and arms and the joints. As a result, muscles and joints—and their attendant smaller structures, the ligaments and tendons—are commonly injured in exercise. Most frequent are knee problems, shinsplints, inflammation of the Achilles tendon, bursitis of the hip, and sore feet. Also common are tennis elbow, painful shoulders, and general muscle aches.

You may have heard (most likely from people who hate to exercise) that exercise predisposes you to permanent joint damage and degen-

133

erative arthritis. This is definitely untrue. In fact, joints are more likely to "rust out" from lack of use than wear out from lots of use. The Arthritis Foundation advises, "Regular exercise is extremely important in controlling some of the symptoms of arthritis. Proper exercises keep joints flexible, build and preserve muscle strength, and help protect joints from further stresses. Improvement in stiff joints or weak muscles may be slow, but those who follow a daily exercise program closely are rewarded with easier movement."

Other causes of pain and discomfort besides injury are external factors. Specifically, these are temperature and humidity. Both extremes, severe cold and dryness or severe heat and high humidity, can induce unpleasant, even health-threatening reactions, especially chilblains and frostbite, dehydration, heat exhaustion, fainting, and heatstroke.

All these injuries and illnesses *can* be prevented by applying some basic principles:

DRESS RIGHT
DRINK UP
WARM UP
COOL DOWN

Dress Right

Before you go outdoors to exercise, find out the temperature and humidity; then dress accordingly. Comfort and safety are individual matters. When some persons exercise, they are very reactive to cold, while others sweat heavily in even mild temperatures. Know yourself, and dress accordingly. If you are just starting to exercise outdoors, dress in layers so that you can peel down as your metabolism heats up. A good rule is to wear one layer less of clothing than you would wear if you were not exercising. After a while, you will pretty well know which combination of clothes is best for you under certain conditions. For example, here is one pattern.

Above 60° F: shorts, light T-shirt
50° F to 60° F: shorts, heavy T-shirt
40° F to 50° F: shorts, light T-shirt, zippered sweat jacket
20° F to 40° F: sweat pants, T-shirt, sweat shirt
0° F to 20° F: sweat pants, T-shirt, sweat shirt, sweat jacket

This pattern of dress indicates what to wear as you leave the house. Then, as you start sweating during exercise, open up clothes or peel them off. A zippered cardigan-style sweat shirt is useful in mildly cool weather because it can be opened to allow some air circulation after you warm up. If you take off the cardigan completely, you might be chilled in your sweat. On the other hand, in warm weather, even a cutoff T-shirt has to be slipped off.

Never, in *any* weather, wear a plastic or rubberized sweat suit. It will induce excessive and dangerous sweating, which can lead to dehydration.

In very cold weather—that is, below freezing—you should be especially attentive to protecting protuberant parts of your body, especially the nose, ears, nipples, penis, fingers, and toes. A protective layer of hand cream helps, as do face masks, a knit hat pulled down over your ears, gloves, heavy socks, and heavy underwear.

In very warm weather, and in heated indoor facilities, you have to dress lightly enough to allow your perspiration to evaporate. If you do indoor chair exercises, dress very lightly because your back and buttocks are covered and will tend to perspire.

If you find yourself sweating excessively at any time, no matter how light or strenuous the exercise, slow down or otherwise cut back on your level of intensity to avoid losing too much fluid from your body.

You also can avoid excess water loss by scheduling your exercise for the more moderate times of the day. In summer, this would be early morning; in winter, later afternoon. You want the cooler, early part of the day in summer, since the hotter afternoon hours cause excessive water loss through perspiration. You want the warmer, later part of the day in winter, since the colder, earlier hours cause excessive water loss through evaporation into the dry air. Also, if the warm environment is indoors, turn down the thermostat an hour or two before you intend to exercise, or open some windows.

What you want to avoid is dehydration, or excess loss of water. It can lead to depletion of blood volume and dangerously high body temperature, which could provoke new or worsen existing health problems.

Remember that your body is a heat machine. It produces basic heat as a by-product of its efforts to keep you alive; it produces excess heat during strenuous physical activity. At the same time, your body works to maintain a constant temperature, which in health varies no more than 1° F from 98.6° F.

When the air around you is dry, your bare skin evaporates moisture, thereby producing cooling. Clothing blocks skin and tends to interfere with evaporative cooling. Also, when the air around you is muggy, the moisture on your skin does not evaporate as readily as when the air is dry. Still, the body pours out sweat in a vain effort to get cooled down.

You can see how the combination of clothes, heat, physical activity, and high humidity works to lower your water level and raise your heat level. Knowing this, you can dress, drink, and plan for a warm environment.

One final thought. Your body can become acclimatized. It takes about two weeks to get used to a warm or cold climate. Now, with heating and air conditioning, hardly anyone in our indoor society really becomes acclimatized to the seasons, living as we do in almost constant temperatures in home, auto, shop, and office.

Drink Up

When it is warm, you have to be sure that you are drinking enough water. There is not much danger of your not getting enough salt. Even if you are on a low-salt diet and are careful and don't add salt to your food, you are eating plenty of salt. You can tell that there is sufficient salt in the U.S. diet by looking at the contents lists that are part of the labels of packaged foods in the United States.

And, while fast foods don't have labels that you can read, they do contain plenty of salt. Food manufacturers and processors say that they add salt to their foods to serve the American palate. Also, salt is added to foods such as bacon and sausage to cure them and to foods such as breads and cakes as essential ingredients. Of course, many foods naturally contain salt, especially vegetables and ocean fish such as tuna and lobster. Furthermore, a well-conditioned body conserves salt and doesn't release as much in perspiration as does a body in poor physical condition.

A good rule to follow is to drink a pint of water about fifteen minutes before you exercise in heat, drink some more during your exercise, and drink lots after.

Warm Up

Any exercise routine, whether done in bed or on an outdoor track, must begin with a warm-up. This is an essential part of the routine, as important as the exercise itself. It prepares your body for the exercise, and unless your body is prepared, exercise may do more harm than good.

Not even teenagers can jump right into an exercise or sport without a warm-up. If their young bodies are not ready, they can suffer many of the same injuries you would suffer if you didn't warm up. But—and this is an important *but*—the older you are, the easier it is for you to be injured because of loss of elasticity of muscle, tendon, and ligament tissue that usually occurs with the years. The corollary is that the older you are, the more important the warm-up is to you. There is an inverse ratio here: as years increase, tolerance to abuse decreases.

You can (as can anyone who exercises) get your cue from professional athletes. At any baseball game, the players warm up before they pitch, throw, bat, or run. So, too, football players, tennis stars, basketball dunkers, hockey hitters, and all kinds of amateur and professional athletes who compete warm up before they spring into action. The warm-up principle applies to everyone who exercises.

One of the main purposes of the warm-up is to increase the blood flow to the muscles. This will provide them with nutrition and oxygen and also raise their temperature 3° F to 5° F. While resting body temperature is 98° F, exercising body temperature is 103° F.

Every warm-up period should last five to ten minutes. This gives your body's circulatory system an opportunity to get ready by opening up the blood vessels that feed into skeletal and heart muscles and gives the metabolic system an opportunity to get ready to meet the demand about to be placed on it. It also prepares the joints for action by increasing their lubrication.

The best warm-up activity is a mild version of the activity that will be your exercise. Dr. Gabe Mirkin explains, "The way you warm up is to use your muscles the same way you're going to use them when you exercise. Calisthenics are a complete waste of time for warming up for other activities. You warm up for bicycling by cycling slowly; you warm up for running by running slowly or walking. You don't warm up for hockey by swimming! So do the activity, but slowly."

While some authorities suggest stretching—lengthening muscle and tendon—as part of the warm-up, Dr. Mirkin warns sedentary older persons against it. "Theoretically, every time you exercise, your muscles are injured because you lose some muscle fibers. The fibers that grow back are the short type. In older persons, these fibers are also brittle. That means that when a sedentary seventy-year-old stretches a tight, exercised muscle, he is liable to tear those new fibers." That certainly will cause discomfort and even pain, which you want to avoid. Middle-aged and older persons who have stayed physically active all their lives can probably get away with some mild warm-up stretching at least until they begin to feel pain (*not* soreness). But if you are a beginner who is just starting to exercise, give warm-up stretching a pass until you are in better physical fitness condition.

This may sound confusing, since this book offers stretching exercises in another chapter. However, those exercises are very mild and intended to increase just your overall flexibility. They are not at all at the level of intensity of warm-up stretches that competitive athletes use, which pull on particular tendons, ligaments, and muscles used in specific exercises and sports. Only if you have continued doing stretching exercises all your life should you stretch in your warm-up routine—and then only gently, without bouncing and without pulling muscles and tendons to their limits.

Cool Down

You yearn for that shower or bath after exercising. Hold it! Don't hurry to the water. Take ten to twenty minutes to let your body get used to its return to the slower pace. The cool-down is as important as the warm-up. You can think of it as the third act of a three-act performance: warm up, exercise, cool down.

The cool-down is important because it permits your body's metabolism to taper down, your muscles to cool off, and both your respiration rate and heartbeat to slow down gradually to normal.

The best cool-down activities, like the best warm-up activities, consist of doing whatever exercise you have been doing, but more slowly and more gently. As with the warm-up, only if you have been doing stretching exercises for as long as you can remember should you do them to cool down.

There is a rule of thumb for determining when you are cooled down enough to take that refreshing bath or shower. You are ready when your skin feels cool and dry to the touch—cool, not cold.

This leads to another particular danger to watch out for—*hypothermia*. Otherwise known as abnormally low body temperature, hypothermia poses a threat to health. It can occur after exercise, when you are sweating, and especially when your clothes are soaking wet. If the ambient air is dry, cold, and moving, your sweat will cool your skin evaporatively so that you lose too much body heat.

The principle is the same as is used in large building air conditioners with water ladders atop the roof. The water that removes the heat from the air circulating inside the building has to get rid of that heat. That is accomplished by having it fall freely down a set of open ladders in the outside air. As the water falls, some of it evaporates into the air; the physical act of evaporating removes the heat from the water. Thus cooled, the water can be circulated through the air-conditioning system to remove yet more heat from the interior of the building.

But you are not a large air conditioner. Your metabolism has wound down, and your body's heat-removal requirements are drastically reduced after exercising. So if you undertake such effective temperature-reducing procedures as a cold shower or lots of iced drinks, you stand the chance of cooling down too fast, which can result in chilling and hypothermia.

To prevent hypothermia, or any chilling after strenuous exercise, remove all your wet clothes and wrap yourself in a warm robe. Take some coffee or other warm beverage, and read the newspaper during the fifteen to twenty minutes your body takes to get back to normal. Keep in mind that your body requires more time to cool down than it does to warm up. Remember, too, that even light activity can fan your metabolic flames so that you sweat. And sweating is the best indication of how warmed up your body is.

These principles of dress, drink, warm-up, and cool-down apply to all kinds of physical activity, and to all levels of intensity. You need to plan not only exercises but also what to do before and after exercising. So, whatever your exercise plan, observe these principles diligently all the time to prevent problems that exercising can bring.

Treating Injuries

The best treatment of injuries is prevention. An old adage, it is still true. Nevertheless, despite your best efforts, injuries will occur. When they do, you should know what to do about those that you can treat, and you should know when to see a doctor for those you cannot treat.

The first part of this chapter dealt with many aspects of prevention of discomfort and pain that can come with exercising—but not all. You'll find other pertinent information on this subject in chapter 15. Your shoes, your swim goggles, the surface you walk on or roll on—all the equipment and materials you use are important. If you are to prevent injuries, you need to pay attention to every consideration about everything you use in exercising and sports.

Another aspect of injury prevention is listening to what your body is telling you. Remember that pain serves a useful purpose; it is a nonverbal message. A message that is fairly quiet and somewhat nagging is likely to mean that some structure has been stressed. A message that is loud and very painful may mean that you have a serious condition that requires medical attention.

A gentle pain tells you to slow down. An example of such a pain is the muscle soreness you may feel the "day after" during the first weeks of your exercise program. Warm baths, massage, and liniment help ease the soreness. Reduced pace and another twenty-four hours help more.

When the pain is severe, your first action should be to stop that particular exercise or activity. If you've pulled a muscle, strained a ligament, or hurt a joint (arthritic or otherwise), stop, and immediately rest the injured part.

The simplest treatment is to elevate the affected area above the level of the heart. This brings gravity in as an ally, to help drain away the excess fluid that accumulates at the site of injury and causes swelling. Elevation thus acts to prevent or minimize swelling.

That is important because the body's natural response to an injury—even though there is no open wound— is to rush blood to the site. But the more blood in the injured area, the greater the swelling, congestion, and pain, and the longer it takes for pain to leave and for healing to finish. Conversely, the less blood in a wound, the less swelling and the shorter the healing time.

If the injury is not serious, the pain may soon subside. If it doesn't, check with your doctor. If he or she permits it, you can try the next stage of injury treatment, cold. You do this by applying ice to the injured area. The benefits of low temperature come from its action on the blood vessels. They contract, thereby decreasing the rate of blood flow to the injured area, and thereby reducing swelling.

Of course, rubbing bare ice on your bare skin will probably hurt. Besides, it's messy. So wrap the ice in cloth such as a towel or washcloth.

One trick is to keep some ice in your home freezer in an empty cottage cheese container. A two-pound container yields about the right size hunk of ice, with a flat surface for applying to muscles in an "ice massage."

Rub the ice pack up and down or in a circular motion on the injured area. This ice massage will cause some discomfort for about three minutes; then numbness will set in. In about fifteen or twenty minutes, the pain will ease (you can figure thirty minutes if you are a large person). You should repeat the ice massage every two hours or so during the acute state or when the pain returns.

While the ice massage works well on flat areas, other surfaces—particularly over foot, knee, hand, and arm injuries—are not as easy to treat this way. They are better treated by immersion. First, wrap the painful part in a plastic bag; then dunk it in an ice-water bath. (Bare skin can be injured in ice water.)

There is a third technique for limiting swelling to an afflicted area, wrapping an elastic bandage tightly about it. This can be combined with cold treatment. In any case, after thirty minutes, unwrap the bandage so the blood can flow again. After fifteen minutes, rewrap. Continue in the same manner for several hours.

Elevation, ice, and bandages are effective ways to treat *sprains,* which result when ligaments (which lash bones of a joint together) are stretched too far or are torn. After three days of ice treatment, switch to heat treatment. Warm baths are the best, but hot compresses work, too. If the pain is sharp, or if, after a week, even moderate pain presists, see a doctor. It might be more serious than a sprain. It could be a *fracture* of a bone, especially a stress fracture; a crack in the bone that was produced when muscles pulled too hard repeatedly; or an early warning of osteoporosis, a condition in which the bone weakens, in part because of loss of calcium. (Getting enough calcium in your diet is one way to prevent osteoporosis. Exercise is another; bones that are used stay strong.)

Muscle cramps can be simple and innocent or complex and dangerous. It all depends on the cause. The most common causes are physical exertion, injury, or strain on the muscle. Less common are nutritional deficiencies of potassium, salt, or magnesium. You can usually prevent potassium-deficiency cramps by eating a potassium-rich banana a day. Salt, as previously mentioned, is abundant in the normal diet. But under conditions of oppressive heat and heavy sweating, it is possible for you to reach a deficient state. In that case, salting your food would be a very good idea. Salt tablets, however, are *not* a good idea, since they produce a great deal of acidity in the stomach and can threaten those persons prone to forming peptic ulcers. Magnesium, too, is important when exercising in hot conditions. It is most abundant in these foods: brussels sprouts; green, leafy vegetables; wheat germ; whole grains; brewer's yeast; beans; and nuts.

Stitches, that sudden pain in the midsection, are produced by a cramp of the diaphragm, the flat muscle that separates the organs of the chest from the organs of the abdomen. A frequent cause of stitches is the very deep breathing that comes with physical exertion, which has the effect of pushing down the lungs and cutting off blood to the diaphragm. Exercising immediately after eating may produce a similar effect by taking blood from the diaphragm.

Recovering from Injury

Aspirin or an aspirin substitute is the strongest kind of drug you should take without a doctor's prescription for an athletic injury—and, even then, only with your doctor's permission, unless, of course, you cannot immediately reach your doctor. While aspirin is safe for most persons, its masking of pain can interfere with the doctor's diagnosis. And always wash down your pills with a full glass of water.

Once the pain of an athletic injury has subsided, you should start gently exercising the injured part, unless your doctor indicates otherwise. The sooner you use this part of your body, the sooner it will get back its strength and flexibility. Remember to exercise moderation as well as your muscles. If you experience any pain, back off. A few isometric exercises without motion may serve as first-phase rehabilitation. Apply only mild pressure for short periods of time.

As your strength returns, start mild exercises that involve motion. Again, use moderation. If appropriate, you might even try some exercises against mild resistance.

If you are careful and consistent, you will find that you will be able to prevent pain and injuries. They usually occur in persons (even professional athletes) who let their guard slip and "forget" to do what they should—properly warm up, for instance. Just remember that no matter your age and activity level, pain and injury are always possible.

Don't let the threat of injury deter you from regular exercising. If you follow the rules with *no exceptions,* you'll enjoy the benefits of exercise for the rest of your life and not have to suffer any pain or injury.

15 Choosing Equipment, Facilities, and Classes

In your enthusiasm to get started and get in shape, you may find many temptations to commit yourself to buying exercise equipment for your home, to taking out a membership in a health club or spa, and to signing up for exercise classes, all of which may be optional to your fitness program. Adding to the pressure is the force of friends and trends. However, before you yield to any or all of these temptations, spend a few minutes considering the benefits and costs and learning how to evaluate equipment, facilities, and experts. And then remind yourself that many good exercises require no outlay of money.

There is a lot of bad exercise equipment screaming to be bought and cheap. There are many clubs and classes that promise much, charge much, and deliver very little. There are a good number of self-proclaimed exercise experts. But there is no certification for any of this. When you are starting out, it's not easy to tell the legitimate from the phony.

Paring it, preening it, pumping it up and pounding it down, the body national is being rejuvenated with a relentless impatience, slimmed with fanatic dedication . . . a wholesale attempt to transform the body is avidly purchased with VISA and MasterCard. The shopping spree is a wild one. The market for all kinds of sport shoes alone has reached $1-billion . . . $240-million for barbells and aerobic dance programs. Health clubs and corporate fitness centers add another $5-billion, sporting togs and gear $8-billion.
—*Time* Magazine

Exercise Equipment

The problem is that there is an abundance—actually an overabundance—of exercise equipment to choose from and to buy. You will find home gyms, exercise cycles, treadmills, rowing machines, trampolines, and all other manner of such equipment at sports stores, at such department stores as Sears, Ward's, and Penney's, and in catalogs from these firms as well as from many other mail-order companies.

Don't be in a rush, despite the advertising, sales, and peer pressures. Have your fitness program planned before you even look for equipment to buy; then buy only if you still feel you *really* need it. When you do look, shop around, ask friends, and become familiar with

143

the kinds and brands of equipment you are considering. Once you make the decision, check prices. Most equipment is discounted, so don't take the list price as the final price. As you will see, this is an expensive area you are getting into. It might pay also to compare the cost of buying equipment against the cost of a membership in a health club that has the equipment you want to use.

Exercise Mat

You can't get more basic than an exercise mat, which is particularly comfortable when you do floor calisthenics. And it is not so expensive, though laying a bed sheet over a carpet serves almost as well.

Skip Rope

Probably the simplest and cheapest piece of equipment (and probably the most impractical at this stage) is rope to use for skipping. You can buy a length of clothesline at a hardware store, buy a skip rope at a toy store, or buy a more serious kind of skip rope at a sporting goods store. If you live where the weather can be nasty and you have to exercise indoors, you will need a room that has a ceiling high enough for the rope to clear as you arch it over your head. In any case, don't start this activity until you are in shape and only then if you have no problems with your feet, ankles, knees, or balance.

Trampoline

A small trampoline is also a rather simple piece of equipment and inexpensive. It serves as a surface upon which you can jog indoors when the weather is bad. This presupposes, of course, that you are already

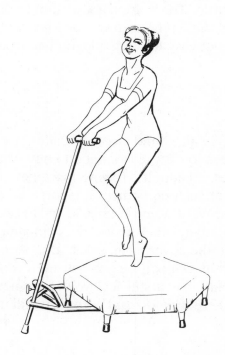

jogging. Select one that is big enough for your stride. Make sure that the equipment has sturdy legs and tough fabric. If you are having trouble with your balance, your back, and/or with joints such as knees, stay away from this one.

Treadmill

If you would rather walk indoors when the weather is inclement, look at a treadmill. It is also good for mild jogging. A basic treadmill is powered only by your feet and kept at an even speed by means of a heavy flywheel. It should have a safety bar at the front and/or sides to hold on to. Some better treadmills have wooden rollers under the tread; these are easier on your feet than metal rollers. The tread should be slip-proof and sturdy. The device probably has a counter to enable you to know the distance you have walked or jogged. It may have an adjustment for increasing the tension and/or an adjustment for increasing or decreasing the angle of steepness, which has the effect of increasing or decreasing the level of work you must do to keep the tread rolling. Fancier treadmills are motorized; they are driven at a speed you select and that you must keep up with. Unless the power switch and speed selector are within your grasp as you are using the device, it could be dangerous. Some of the higher-priced treadmills also have electronic readouts. Because of the variation in complexity, treadmill prices range from hundreds to thousands of dollars.

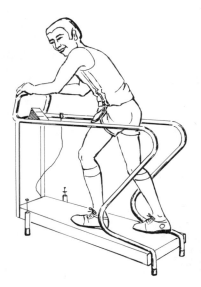

Bicycle

If you want to ride your bicycle indoors, get a stationary stand to place it on. It's not a fancy arrangement, and there are no razzle-dazzle electronic readouts; but it works, and it is cheap. Just make sure that the one you buy is sturdy enough to hold you and your bike. Stands are often listed in catalogs and not shown in stores because retailers would rather sell the higher-priced exercise, or stationary, cycles. The most basic of these cycles is a stand with a bicycle seat and pedals that are connected to a single wheel, the tension of which you can adjust to increase or decrease your work load. Better models allow you to pedal forward and backward and thus exercise muscles on the front as well as the back of the leg. Also important is a range of adjustments of the seat to fit your height and leg length. Even basic cycles have a speedometer and an odometer so you can assess the level of your effort and the distance you have traveled. Fancier ones have electronic readouts linked to microprocessors to let you know all this (as though you had lost touch with the feelings in your muscles and lungs!) as well as how many calories you have just burned. Do *not* (I repeat *not*) buy a cycle that is powered by a motor. That is a waste of money because such machines do the work that you are supposed to do. Also, they can be dangerous.

Rowing Machine

A rowing machine looks better than it actually is as a piece of exercise equipment. It is what it sounds like, a device that enables you to simulate on land the actions of rowing a dinghy in the water. Unlike a dinghy bench, the rowing machine seat slides forward and back. The pressure required to pull the "oars" should be adjustable. Some rowing machines also have adjustable sliding pressure so that the seat slides with more or less difficulty, as you prefer.

Exercise cycles and rowing machines are both deficient in that they exercise only one part of the body. In the case of the cycle, it is the lower body; in the case of the rowing machine, it is the upper body. By using both in your exercising program, you can do most of your body some good.

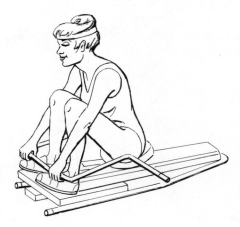

Skiing Machine

By contrast, a cross-country skiing machine exercises both the upper and lower parts of your body—if skiing is an activity you can and like to pursue. Unfortunately, there are only a few models to choose from.

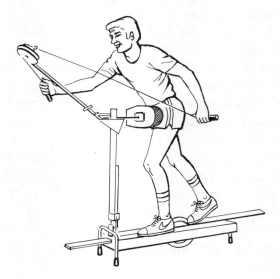

Weights

You may not think that you would want to lift weights—push iron—at this stage of your life. Maybe you will decide not to, but don't completely close your mind to the idea. Of course you're not trying to build your muscle mass into what is required for a Mr. or Mrs. America, but that is not all that weight training is good for. Weights can be a very good way to build muscle strength, especially if you are chair-bound. Free (not attached to any device or wall) weights such as barbells and dumbbells are the best buy and the easiest to store. Exercise benches and weight machines offer more flexibility of use. Of course, with more and more features come higher and higher prices, up into the thousands.

Ys, Js, Health Clubs, and Spas

If you are just starting your exercise program, you may want to consider going to some sort of facility where there are "experts" to guide you, machines and perhaps a sauna and whirlpool to use, and others in your situation so you won't have the feeling of being left on your own. Many people find motivation in the presence of others who are sweating and grunting in efforts to improve their physical condition. Also, if you want to include swimming in your exercise plan and want to swim year-round, you may need an indoor pool.

The only way you will know whether a facility suits you is to visit it and talk to the staff. Even better, many exercise organizations offer a free visit for people who are considering joining. It doesn't hurt to ask about a free visit when you phone for other information.

Before you commit lots of money to private clubs and spas, look at your community resources. Investigate the "Y" (Young Men's Christian Association, or YMCA; Young Women's Christian Association, or YWCA; Young Men's and Young Women's Hebrew Association, or YM/YWHA) or the "J" (Jewish Community Center, or JCC), the general community center, the park district, the local college, the senior adult center, and other public facilities. You may be surprised at how well equipped and staffed these facilities are. And the fees will likely be much lower than those at private health clubs. Again, assess what you want for your body, and then list and order your priorities.

If you check out a health club, you may find a very commercial exercise salon when you arrive. There are people who are put off from health clubs because of the high-pressure sales tactics so many of them use. You may not be, if that is what you expected. Your decision should be based on a simple analysis of what you get for what you pay. That means separating your feelings from the data. Such separations are not always easy to accomplish.

The following checklist may prove helpful.

Checklist

1. What is the facility's experience? That is, how long has it been in the community, and what is its track record? Do you know anyone who recommends it? Do you know (or can you find out) anything about the background of the people who own and/or run it?

2. Was everything promised and everything stated by a salesperson put in writing?

3. How much time do you have to consider the terms of the contract before signing?

4. Is there a trial period so that you can be sure about the facility before you sign any membership application?

5. May you take a class and a workout before signing?

6. How are the fees paid? Monthly? To whom are they paid—to the club or spa, or to a bank or loan company?

7. Can you afford the membership fee?

8. Are there add-on charges or special fees for any activities or classes? Is there a rental charge for the use of any of the equipment?

9. Can you get a prorated refund if you become ill, are injured, move away, or are unable otherwise to use the facility before your membership expires?

10. If the facility is part of a chain, are there reciprocal privileges at other locations?

11. Is the facility convenient to your workplace or your home?

12. What is the place like during busy times? Is it clean? well maintained? not too crowded? Is the equipment in good condition? Are there adequate locker room and shower facilities?

13. How good are the teaching and supervisory staffs?

14. Are there equal facilities and equal schedule times available for men and women?

There is some good advice from the Federal Trade Commission concerning private clubs. It is in *Health Spas: Exercise Your Rights,* which you can obtain free from the Bureau of Consumer Protection, Federal Trade Commission, 600 E. Street, NW, Washington, DC 20580. The leaflet explains regulations issued by the commission (FTC) as a means of handling the issues raised in many complaints it has received.

Among the regulations is a required three-day cooling-off period to enable the new spa member to have an attorney go over the contract or other papers and to allow the member to change his or her mind for any reason and get the down payment back.

You should know that in some states such establishments are required to post bond and place money in escrow to be available to repay unsatisfied customers or members who are left without a health club when it goes out of business.

In any case, don't let yourself be rushed into signing anything, even with the lure of the great discount that is being offered only during "this" period of time and which is about to expire. Also heed the following:

- Make sure all promises are in writing.

- Make sure that your total membership fee and other fees are listed, as well as the method and timing of your payment.

● Make sure that all interest charged to you is stated, as well as whether or not you are in fact securing a bank loan to pay the fees.

Spas are another story. You know when you consider a spa that it will cost you plenty. In exchange for the high price tag, you will be pampered and coddled. Exercise and dieting will seem luxurious. The problem with any spa—whether nearby, at the other end of the continent, or on a sunny Caribbean isle—is that the luxury and the wonderment are so temporary. *If*—and that is a big *if*—you can establish good exercising habits that carry over to your regular routine back home, the spa visit will accomplish something toward your fitness goal. More usually, that doesn't happen. Instead, you are likely to revert to your old ways when you reenter the familiar hometown environment.

Classes

Dr. Kenneth H. Cooper, the founder of aerobics, observes, "There are a lot of people leading aerobic dancing and other exercise classes who are not qualified in any way to lead them. This can particularly be dangerous for the sedentary woman past fifty who walks into the class for the first time, is given minimal instructions as to what to do, and tries to keep up with other class members—she is intimidated if she doesn't. Intimidation can push her to the point where she will exercise a whole lot more than she should, especially on her first day." For reasons specified in previous chapters, no one should plunge right into exercising, especially after years of no exercising. Dr. Cooper continues, "While I've said 'woman,' this applies to men, as well. I've seen patients who were pushed so hard and their heart rates were so excessive that they might have died right on the exercise floor. That's the kind of problem that can happen when people who have never exercised enroll in exercise classes led by instructors not adequately trained. That's why I feel that a certification program is certain to come in the not-too-distant future."

Dr. Cooper voices a concern that other exercise authorities have also expressed—anyone can proclaim himself or herself an exercise instructor with impunity. Obviously, you can have confidence in following a leader who is qualified.

How do you know whether the leader is qualified? Here are three ways to get answers.

1. If the exercise classes are held at a Y, a community center, or your local college, you reasonably can expect a high level of competence in the exercise leaders.

2. You can ask your private physician for recommended exercise classes.

3. You can ask for the credentials of the leader of any class you want to join. You can expect the leader to be a graduate of an accredited program of physical education, physical rehabilitation, physical therapy, or physical medicine. Some of these specialists, such as fitness instructors and physical therapists, are certified. (In November 1984, the American College of Sports Medicine announced that it had started developing certification for fitness instructors in three areas: dance-exercise, military and law enforcement, and business and industry.)

Think Before You Spend

As you can see, there is a good deal to consider when you reach the point of spending money for an exercise program. As in starting any new program, you have to learn everything you can about it. The time you spend in educating yourself is a good and necessary investment.

Once you have explored and investigated equipment, facilities, classes, and leaders, you should sit down and go over the data you have accumulated and make your decision without sales or peer pressures. It's your body and your health, so you should be the only one making decisions about yourself. The only person you might ask for help is your physician. In any case, try to spend the minimum amount of money, and exercise at a maximum of convenience to yourself.

16 Sports for Seniors

I would strongly urge every American to find a sport that he or she enjoys. Those who do so will be making a sound investment in future health and happiness.
—Ronald Reagan, President of the United States

Once you are in shape, you may want to consider participating in sports. It could be a game or sport that you participated in years ago, such as softball or basketball, or it could be a new one, such as tennis or racquetball. It could even be a competitive sport, such as Master swimming.

You may be surprised to learn that there are many thousands of persons your age who participate regularly in Masters events sponsored by the Amateur Athletic Union (AAU). Masters competitions are held in just about all athletic events and are held locally, statewide, regionally, and nationally. They are open to all persons who are twenty-five years of age and older. And the "older" is open.

Masters athletes compete in each event against Masters athletes of their own sex and approximate age. Thus men aged fifty-five to fifty-nine swim the freestyle against one another, and women sixty to sixty-four swim the breaststroke against one another.

You don't have to go as far as competing, but it should give you pleasure to realize that you can now consider such possibilities. And, if you do participate, you will find that the right sport will help maintain and even improve your physical fitness, as well as your mental health. It will also help you relax.

This chapter presents a range of sports activities for you to consider, along with some addresses to which you can write for more information and membership applications. In addition, many states hold Senior Olympics every year. Among them are Illinois, Indiana, Rhode Island, and Virginia. For more information on these events, look up AAU (Amateur Athletic Union) in the phone book. Or you can write

153

to the following, which are good sources of general information on sports:

> President's Council on Physical Fitness and Sports
> 450 5th Street, NW
> Washington, DC 20001

> American Athletic Union of the U.S.
> 3400 W. 86th Street
> Indianapolis, IN 46268
> Mason Bell, Executive Director
> (1-317-872-2900)

> National Senior Sports Association
> 317 Cameron Street
> Alexandria, VA 22314
> Eugene J. Skora, Executive Director
> (1-703-549-6711)

> Senior Sports International, Inc.
> Suite 360
> 5670 Wilshire Boulevard
> Los Angeles, CA 90036

The best sport for fitness is one that you enjoy, that requires sustained effort, and that challenges you. If you are in top shape, the sport should also challenge your endurance and help your cardiovascular health.

As with the exercises you have mastered, you should start a sport reasonably slowly. Don't rush in and think you will be a champion right away. Mastering any activity takes time and effort. You can be a champion, but that takes as much patience as fervor. It also takes time in another dimension—solid blocks of dedicated time in your weekly schedule.

Any sport can substitute for your usual workout if it is at the same level of physical intensity.

What follows is a list of sports and games for you to consider. While the list is not all-inclusive, it should offer some possibilities for you. With each sport or game is an evaluation based on fitness.

Baseball/Softball

The versions of softball that use a larger ball—a twelve-inch or sixteen-inch—are the most practical. At best, it is a low-activity game, even for the pitcher. For every other member of the team, the action is sporadic, amounting to running for a ball or a base. Most localities have leagues for seniors. (Amateur Softball Association, 2801 NE 50th Street, RR 4, Box 385, Oklahoma City, OK 73111)

Basketball

Even shooting baskets in your driveway will get you winded rather quickly, which is one reason this is not recommended for persons who are out of shape. But if you are in top shape and have no hip, knee, or foot problems, the running and jumping are vigorous enough to be an excellent endurance and cardiovascular sport. If you want to play basketball, play with contemporaries who are in as good shape as you; don't play against sixteen-year-olds! This sport is particularly good for slimming, endurance, and cardiovascular goals.

Bowling

Sociable but not vigorous, bowling is murder on bad backs because you are lifting fifteen pounds or so on one side and walking and bending with the weight. Physically, it helps you in balance and coordination and develops the muscles of one arm. There are leagues for seniors. (American Bowling Congress, 5301 South 76th Street, Greendale, WI 53129; 1-414-421-6400; Roger Tessman, Executive Secretary. Also, National Senior Sports Association, noted on page 154.)

Cycling

This is a great way to use those big muscles in your legs and to exercise vigorously for cardiovascular endurance and muscle strength. If balance is not a problem, you can get outdoors, in fresh air, and enjoy scenery as you exercise. If balance and/or weather is a problem, you can work out on a stationary bicycle indoors. The problem outdoors can be traffic; the problem indoors can be boredom. Solve the former problem by wearing a helmet and observing all traffic laws, rules, and courtesies. Solve the latter problem by reading a book, listening to the stereo, watching TV, or pedaling with a pal. There are cycling competitions for older persons. (United Cycling Federation, USCF Building 4, 1750 East Boulder Street, Colorado Springs, CO 80909)

Football/Soccer

This is not the kind of activity associated with seniors, but remember the Kennedy family's games, in which all ages (and both sexes) played. Of course, the college or professional kind, which stops a runner by tackling, is unsuitable. But touch or flag football should be OK. Even more suitable is soccer, which requires more consistent running. Both are best played outdoors. Neither football nor soccer should be considered if you have hip, knee, or foot problems. Also, don't try to play with a team of teenagers, no matter how great you were "back then."

Golf

A great way to get outdoors and be in fresh air amid greenery, golf is a low-intensity sport. In terms of physical activity, an eighteen-hole game is equivalent to a casual stroll of about three miles. However, if you walk, you are likely to be alone; most golfers use motorized carts. Be sure you limber up your arms, shoulders, and back before you play so you won't suffer the bad effects of the sudden swing you take to drive the ball into the air. There are tournaments for seniors, including the national Senior Open, Senior Amateur, and Senior Women's Amateur. (United States Golf Association, Golf House, Far Hills, NJ 07931; also, National Senior Sports Association, noted on page 154.)

Field Hockey

Not popular in all sections of the United States, this is a sport that knows no age divisions. You need good running legs. (Field Hockey Association of America, 1750 East Boulder Street, Colorado Springs, CO 80909)

Horseback Riding

Like golf, this is a great way to get outdoors and inhale fresh air. Unlike golf, riding can be done in all seasons. It requires skill and some leg strength, but it is not an endurance activity. If you have balance problems, this is not for you.

Racket Games

Once the question Tennis, anyone? was greeted with a smile and inaction. Today it is answered loudly and affirmatively. Also popular are other sports that require rackets (or racquets), including table tennis (Ping-Pong), badminton, and the various versions of squash—paddleball, racquetball, and handball. (Handball is included, though no racket is used, because it is so similar.) The games that use a net are mildly active—more so for singles, less so for doubles. The games played against the floor and walls of a small room are vigorous. All have senior tournaments. Take your pick. (U.S. Tennis Association, 51 East 42nd Street, New York, NY 10017; U.S. Handball Association, 4101 Dempster Street, Skokie, IL 60076; U.S. Racquetball Association, 4101 Dempster Street, Skokie, IL 60076; U.S. Squash Racquets Association, Inc., 211 Ford Road, Bala Cynwyd, PA 19004)

Rowing

Sculling, the more formal name for rowing or crewing, is a national Master sport. In competition it can indeed be vigorous, though exercise is limited to the arms and upper body. (National Association of Amateur Oarsmen, 4 Boathouse Row, Philadelphia, PA 19130)

Running

If you like to run, there are competitions all over the place—from one-mile runs to twenty-seven-mile marathons, from community meets to Senior Olympics. These attract people of all ages, including yours. Aside from needing good feet, good knees, good hips, good lungs, and a good heart, you need the will to train. (50+ Runners Association, PO Box D, Stanford, CA 94305; 1-415-497-6254; Dr. Peter Wood, Executive Officer. Also, American Running & Fitness Association, 2420 K Street, NW, Washington, DC 20037; 1-202-965-3430; Liz Elliott, Executive Director. Also, AAU, noted on page 154.)

Skating

Skating is not an activity to start unless you have perfect balance, but if you have been skating all your life, or for many years, and have good balance and strong ankles, you might consider competing on shoe wheels. It can be vigorous and good for both the cardiovascular system and endurance. (U.S. Amateur Confederation of Roller Skating, 7700 A Street, PO Box 83067, Lincoln, NE 68501) Less popular, but equally invigorating is ice skating.

Swimming

There are frequent local, statewide, and regional meets and a national meet for Masters (above the age of twenty-five) in what is probably the most popular sport for seniors. To be a Masters swimmer, you have to be willing to train regularly in this most all-around sport. (U.S. Masters Swimming, PO Box 5039, Sun City, FL 33570)

Tennis

If you have good knees and stamina, tennis is a vigorous sport—singles more than doubles. Like volleyball (see page 158), it has intensified from the gentle lawn sport of your youth to the fast, competitive game you now see on TV. Of course, your playing will be somewhere in between. (National Senior Sports Association, noted on page 154.)

Volleyball

Volleyball is fast becoming one of the world's favorite competitive sports. No longer the gentle lawn game at picnics, it has grown into a vigorous game that tries the jumping and spiking ability and physical endurance of its players at all ages. You do need good feet, good ankles, good knees, and a sporting heart to succeed. There are plenty of senior teams and tournaments around. (U.S. Volleyball Association, 1750 East Boulder Street, Colorado Springs, CO 80909)

Yachting

This is a sport that knows no age; in fact, the best sailors are more likely to have more years than less. It is not physically vigorous unless you work the sails alone or climb the mast. There are races regularly in every body of water in every class of boat, weather permitting. (Inter-Lake Yachting Association, PO Box 435, Vermilion, OH 44089)

17 Go for It!

If we didn't have habits, we could not function properly. . . . If you can ride a bike, you do it by habit without thinking. If you swim, you do it by habit without thinking. When you read, you do it by habit without thinking about the alphabet and the sounds and meanings of each of the 26 letters.
—Richard Stiller, Habits

The hardest part about starting a new program is starting.

But the only way to get started is to start.

Trite as both of these statements are, they are true. The purpose of this chapter is to help you overcome your inertia if you have not started exercising, to get you started in an exercising program, and to keep you exercising.

This book's advice and instructions do you no good if they are only read; they have to be applied. To repeat a point made earlier: No one can do the exercise for you; you must do it yourself. So, stop merely thinking about your exercise program and start it. *Now!*

Getting Started

Here are three steps to get you started.

1. Form a small exercise group with relatives, friends, or acquaintances, or look for such a group to join. It's more than, Misery loves company. Group support works as well or better for exercisers as it does for dieters. It's the beginning of a support system for persons like yourself who can help others out—complimenting one another when progress is made, supporting one another when motivation wanes. A group of half a dozen is about the right size. You have to be realistic and face the fact that while you will be loyal, not everyone else will come every time. Some may be sick; some may be out of town; some may even drop out. If any of the others belong to exercise groups, commercial or otherwise, you will probably be invited as a guest. That will expand your opportunities for exercise. Commercial or community exercise classes and groups can be a fine way to get started exercising and to keep with it. But heed chapter 15's cautions about the qualifications of the exercise leader and its suggestions on ways to resist the high-pressure pitch.

2. Choose a sport, such as volleyball, or other regular activity you like, such as walking, rather than one you dislike, such as jogging, but think may be good for you. If you apply the saying, Nothing succeeds like success, you will succeed with an activity you like because that is bound to be an activity you succeed in. Why fight it?

3. Realize that in starting your exercise program, you are starting a habit—a good habit. Don't dwell on having to break bad old habits. That's an unproductive direction for your energy and an attitude that does no good. There are two important premises in starting a habit and maintaining it that you should know and apply. They are the two Rs. Learn them and make them your motto. They are *reinforcement* and *repetition.*

Reinforcement, or reward, is the good feeling you get from accomplishing something. You should associate a good feeling with exercise in order to develop it into a habit. It is the same as developing other habits. Since you liked the taste, texture, and aroma of foods and the way food ended the feeling of hunger, you developed the habit of eating regularly. If you liked the feeling of satisfaction and release with coitus, you made sex a habit. If you liked the social approval you got when you lost fifty pounds, you kept your weight off. And you were rewarded every time you ate or had sex or as long as you kept trim. Those rewards reinforced your habit, strengthened it. That's how reinforcement works.

That great feeling of pleasant tiredness and relaxation after exercising, which you get no other way, could be a form of reinforcement. So could the admiration from family and friends about how good you look. Best of all reinforcements, though, is the functional fitness you will achieve—the ability to do what you want, at last.

Repetition increases the strength of the habit. As repetitions add up, they require less and less effort, but also have less effect. That means you must be especially diligent at the beginning and repeat your exercise program day after day in order for the habit to get a good start. This is crucial at the beginning and merely important later on, after the exercise program becomes a habit.

Richard Stiller, who wrote the book *Habits,* noted "I can remember without effort my Army serial number from 30 years ago, but I cannot remember the telephone number or even the street address of the house I lived in less than 10 years ago. The Army drilled us so that memory of our serial numbers became fixed by habit, and that memory has never left me. . . . It used reinforcement [you got a pass to go to town if you learned] and repetition [you had to repeat your serial number any time an officer stopped you, and before you could eat or go to the toilet]."

Restarting Your Exercise Program

Unfortunately, about half of all those who start an exercise program eventually drop it. Is that what happened to your last exercise program? And the one before that? In a way, staying on an exercise program is like staying on a cigarette-quitting program. It's easy; you may have done it a dozen times before!

So, here are three tips on what to do and think in order to stay with your exercise habit.

1. **Have the right attitude.** If you have been off your exercise program for any reason, merely consider it a lapse, or an interruption, not a falling away. Those interruptions might be caused by a cold or other illness, by bad weather, by a holiday or vacation, or by an unaccountable lapse of motivation. OK, it's over. Pick yourself up, and get started again. When you reenter your program, drop back a level on the exercise intensity, since you will probably have lost a notch or two of fitness.

2. **Be proud.** That wonderful self-esteem you get from functional fitness is good enough to flaunt. You don't have to shout it on street corners, but when people ask why you look so young, be proud when you tell them about your exercise program. That pride will get you back on the track. Keep yourself in the program by doing the physical thing whenever you can. For instance, park your car at the far, not close, end of the parking lot. Take the stairs instead of the elevator whenever you can. Your less-fit friends will admire you greatly for it. Their admiration will send you back to the pool or the walking path and keep you there.

3. **Stay motivated.** If you have had a relapse, remember your motivation for starting your exercise program. If you are like most adult exercisers, your motivation was to do more and feel less fatigued. And you wanted to look better. Thanks to your exercise program, you have been doing more and are feeling less fatigued than you have in years. And you look better, too. If you don't get back on the fitness program, you will certainly lose all your gains and slide back to not being able to do as many things as you like or to do them as well.

New World

Being functionally fit can open a whole new world for you. Those years you've accumulated are only numbers. Being fit, you can do things and get around. You can break the stereotype of adults after middle age.

But you can achieve even more by working on your fitness habits and by pushing your body to do more. And you *can* do more. Just go for it!

Bibliography

You may want to look up more information from books, pamphlets, and articles quoted in the text. Here are citations for the sources quoted.

Adult Physical Fitness—A Program for Men and Women. Administration on Aging. Washington, D.C.: U.S. Government Printing Office, 1980.

"America Shapes Up." *Time,* 118(2 Nov. 1981): 94–106.

Aqua Dynamics. Washington, D.C.: The President's Council on Physical Fitness and Sports, n.d.

Basic Exercises for People Over 60. Washington, D.C.: National Association for Human Development, 1976.

Berland, Theodore. *The Fitness Fact Book.* New York: Enterprise Publications, 1980; New American Library, 1981.

———. *Rating the Diets.* Skokie, Ill.: Publications International, 1986.

Björntorp, Per. "Interrelation of Physical Activity and Nutrition on Obesity." In *Diet and Exercise: Synergism in Health Maintenance* edited by Philip L. White and Therese Mondeika. Chicago: American Medical Association, 1982.

Church, Charles Frederick, and Helen Nichols Church. *Food Values of Portions Commonly Used. Bowes and Church.* 11th ed. Philadelphia: J.B. Lippincott Co., 1970.

Cooper, Kenneth H. *Aerobics.* New York: Bantam Books, 1968.

———. *The New Aerobics.* New York: Bantam Books, 1970.

———. *The Aerobics Program for Total Well-Being.* New York: Bantam Books, 1982.

Corbin, Charles B.; Linus J. Dowell; Ruth Lindsey; and Homer Tolson. *Concepts in Physical Education.* Dubuque, Iowa: Wm. C. Brown Co., 1982.

Corbin, David E., and Josie Metal-Corbin. *Reach for It! A Handbook of Exercise and Dance Activities for Older Adults.* Dubuque, Iowa: eddie bowers, 1983.

Council on Scientific Affairs. "Exercise Programs for the Elderly." *Journal of the American Medical Association* 252 (July 1984): 544–546.

DeVries, Herbert A. *Physiology of Exercise for Physical Education and Athletics.* 3rd ed. Dubuque, Iowa: Wm. C. Brown Co., 1980.

DeVries, Herbert A., with Diane Hales. *Fitness after 50.* New York: Charles Scribner's Sons, 1982.

Exercise Activity for People Over 60. Washington, D.C.: National Association for Human Development, 1977.

Exercise, Diet and Nutrition for People Over 60. Washington, D.C.: National Association for Human Development, 1978.

Fahey, Thomas D. "What to Do About Athletic Injuries." In *Guide to Fitness After Fifty* edited by Raymond Harris and Lawrence J. Frankel. New York: Plenum Press, 1978.

The Fitness Challenge . . . in the Later Years. Washington, D.C.: U.S. Government Printing Office, 1975.

Folan, Lilias M. *Lilias, Yoga, and Your Life.* New York: Collier Books, 1981.

Frankel, Lawrence J., and Betty Byrd Richard. *Be Alive as Long as You Live.* New York: Lippincott & Crowell, 1980.

Harris, Raymond, and Lawrence J. Frankel, eds. *Guide to Fitness After Fifty.* New York: Plenum Press, 1978.

Holloszy, John O. "Exercise, Health, and Aging: A Need for More Information." *Medicine and Science in Sports and Exercise* 15(1983): 1–5.

Jacobson, Edmund. *Progressive Relaxation.* Chicago: The University of Chicago Press, 1968.

———. *You Must Relax.* 5th ed. New York: McGraw-Hill Book Co., 1976.

———. "The Origins and Development of Progressive Relaxation." *Journal of Behavior Therapy and Experimental Psychiatry.* 8(1977): 119–123.

Johnson, Harry J. *Creative Walking for Physical Fitness.* New York: Grosset & Dunlap, 1970.

Join the Active People Over 60! Washington, D.C.: National Association for Human Development, 1976.

Konishi, Frank. *Exercise Equivalents of Food.* Carbondale, Ill.: Southern Illinois University Press, 1973.

Kuntzleman, Charles T. *The Exerciser's Handbook.* New York: David McKay Co., 1978.

———. *Your Active Way to Weight Control.* Clinton, Iowa: 1980.

Kusinitz, Ivan; Morton Fine and the editors of Consumer Reports Books. *Physical Fitness for Practically Everybody.* Mount Vernon, N.Y.: Consumers Union, 1983.

Lamb, Lawrence E. "Stay Youthful and Fit." In *Statements on Physical Fitness for Older Persons.* Washington, D.C.: National Association for Human Development, 1976.

Leslie, David K., and John W. McLure. *Exercises for the Elderly.* Des Moines, Iowa: Iowa Commission on the Aging, 1975.

Mirkin, Gabe, and Marshall Hoffman. *The Sportsmedicine Book.* Boston: Little, Brown & Co., 1978.

Moderate Exercises for People Over 60. Washington, D.C.: National Association for Human Development, 1976.

Myers, Clayton R. *The Official YMCA Physical Fitness Handbook.* New York: Popular Library, 1975.

Nutritive Value of American Foods in Common Units. Agriculture Handbook No. 456. Washington, D.C.: U.S. Government Printing Office, 1975.

Nutritive Value of Foods. Home and Garden Bulletin No. 72. rev. Washington, D.C.: U.S. Government Printing Office, 1977.

Pep Up Your Life: A Fitness Book for Seniors. Hartford, Conn.: The Travelers Insurance Companies, n.d. (Written in cooperation with the President's Council on Physical Fitness and Sports.)

Recommended Dietary Allowances. 9th ed. Washington, D.C.: National Academy of Sciences, 1980.

Spackman, Robert R., Jr. *Conditioning for Senior Citizens.* Murphysboro, Ill.: Schwebel Printing, 1981.

Statements on Physical Fitness for Older Persons. Washington, D.C.: National Association for Human Development, 1976.

Stiller, Richard. *Habits.* Nashville, Tenn.: Thomas Nelson, Inc., 1977.

A Synopsis of the National Conference on Fitness and Aging, September 10–11, 1981, Shoreham Hotel, Washington, D.C. Washington, D.C.: The President's Council on Physical Fitness and Sports, n.d.

Vodak, Paul. *Exercise: The Why and the How.* Palo Alto, Cal.: Bull Publishing Co., 1980.

Index

About the Author

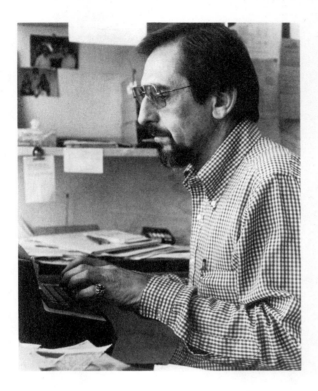

Theodore Berland has served as a writer on health and fitness for The University of Chicago, Michael Reese Hospital and Medical Center, Rush-Presbyterian-St. Luke's Medical Center, and numerous health associations. He is past president of the American Medical Writers Association and of the Society of Midland Authors. He is a Life Member of the National Association of Science Writers. This is Berland's sixteenth book. He has also written more than 300 articles for newspapers and magazines—some of which won awards—and for six years wrote a syndicated column on dieting.

A 1950 journalism graduate of the University of Illinois (Urbana), Berland obtained his Master's degree in Sociology at The University of Chicago in 1972 and took additional graduate work at Bowling Green State University, Ohio. He has been on the faculties of Bowling Green; the University of Wisconsin-Milwaukee; Columbia College, Chicago, where he was chairman of the Department of Journalism; and Grand Valley State College, Michigan, where he is Associate Professor of Communications.

A popular speaker on fitness, Berland exercises at the high-intensity level. During most weeks, he swims a mile three times and jogs five miles three times. During the summer he enjoys sailing his Sunfish off the beach near Chicago, where he and his wife live. They have three grown children: two daughters who have graduated from college and started careers and a son who is in his senior year in college.

PLANNING YOUR RETIREMENT HOUSING
by Michael Sumichrast, Ronald G. Shafer, and Marika Sumichrast
673-24810-0 $8.95

POLICY WISE, The Practical Guide to Insurance Decisions for Older Consumers
by Nancy H. Chasen
673-24806-2 $5.95

SUNBELT RETIREMENT
by Peter A. Dickinson
673-24832-1 $11.95

SURVIVAL HANDBOOK FOR WIDOWS (and for relatives and friends who want to understand)
by Ruth J. Loewinsohn
673-24820-8 $5.95

TRAVEL EASY, The Practical Guide for People Over Fifty
by Rosalind Massow
673-24817-8 $8.95

WHAT TO DO WITH WHAT YOU'VE GOT, The Practical Guide to Money Management in Retirement
by Peter Weaver and Annette Buchanan
673-24805-4 $7.95

YOUR VITAL PAPERS LOGBOOK
673-24833-X $4.95

For complete information write: AARP Books, 1900 East Lake Avenue, Glenview, IL 60025 or contact your local bookstore.

Prices subject to change.